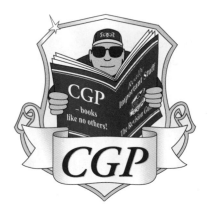

GCSE History is always topical with CGP...

"Medicine in Britain, c1250-Present" can be a gruesome part of Edexcel GCSE History, but this CGP Topic Guide will help you answer exam questions with surgical precision.

It's packed with crystal-clear revision notes explaining the whole topic, plus plenty of useful activities, sample answers, exam tips and exam-style questions. You'll never get sick of it!

CGP — still the best! ☺

Our sole aim here at CGP is to produce the highest quality books — carefully written, immaculately presented and dangerously close to being funny.

Then we work our socks off to get them out to you — at the cheapest possible prices.

Published by CGP

Editors:
Izzy Bowen, Andy Cashmore, Robbie Driscoll, Catherine Heygate, Holly Robinson

Contributors:
Rachel Ellis-Lomas and Paddy Gannon

With thanks to Sarah Elsdon and Louise McEvoy for the proofreading.
With thanks to Jan Greenway and Emily Smith for the copyright research.

Acknowledgements:

Cover image: Florence Nightingale. The Lady with the Lamp, visiting the sick soldiers in hospital,
Jackson, Peter (1922-2003) / Private Collection / © Look and Learn / Bridgeman Images

With thanks to Alamy for permission to use the images on pages 5, 69 and 84.

With thanks to Mary Evans Picture Library for permission to use the images on pages 6, 12, 18, 22, 26, 32, 40, 50, 52 and 58.

Extract on page 69: War Diaries: A Nurse at the Front - The First World War Diaries of Sister Edith Appleton, edited by Ruth Cowen
Text copyright © Dick Robinson and Imperial War Museums 2012, reproduced by kind permission of Simon & Schuster UK Ltd

Trench diagram on page 70 © Crown Copyright. Contains public sector information licensed under the Open Government Licence v3.0
http://www.nationalarchives.gov.uk/doc/open-government-licence/version/3/

Trench map of Hill 60 in April 1917 on page 70. Reproduced with permission from the National Library of Scotland.

With thanks to the Imperial War Museum for permission to use the image on page 71.

Extract on page 73: Reproduced with permission of Curtis Brown Group Ltd, London on behalf of the Estate of R C Sherriff.
Copyright Notice © R C Sherriff, 1996.

Extract on page 75 reproduced courtesy of Queen Square Archives

Extract on page 76: From War Diary of the 10th Canadian Battalion, April 1915, ref. WO 95/3770, National Archives, Kew, Surrey, England

Extract on page 76: Bowlby A. The Bradshaw Lecture on Wounds in War. British Medical Journal. 1915;2(2869):913-921.

Extract on page 77 and Source A on page 81 from the National Archives: contains public sector information licensed under the Open Government Licence v3.0
http://www.nationalarchives.gov.uk/doc/open-government-licence/version/3/

Source B on page 82: © 2007 http://chestofbooks.com/

ISBN: 978 1 78908 289 0
Printed by Elanders Ltd, Newcastle upon Tyne.
Clipart from Corel®

Contents

Exam Hints and Tips

You'll have to take three papers in Edexcel GCSE History. This book will help you to prepare for Paper 1.

You will take 3 Papers altogether

1) Paper 1 is 1 hour 15 minutes long. It's worth 52 marks — 30% of your GCSE. This paper will be divided into 2 sections:
   - Section A: Historic Environment.
   - Section B: Thematic Study.

> This book covers the Thematic Study Medicine in Britain, c.1250-present and the Historic Environment The British Sector of the Western Front, 1914-1918.

2) Paper 2 is 1 hour 45 minutes long. It's worth 64 marks — 40% of your GCSE. This paper will be divided into two question and answer booklets:
   - Booklet P: Period Study.
   - Booklet B: British Depth Study.

> It's really important that you make sure you know which topics you're studying for each paper.

3) Paper 3 is 1 hour 20 minutes long. It's worth 52 marks — 30% of your GCSE. This paper will be divided into 2 sections, both about a Modern Depth Study:
   - Section A: 2 questions, one of which is based on a source.
   - Section B: A four-part question based on 2 sources and 2 interpretations.

Remember these Tips for Approaching the Questions

Organise your Time in the exam

1) The more marks a question is worth, the longer your answer should be.
2) Don't get carried away writing loads for a question that's only worth four marks — you'll need to leave time for the higher mark questions.

> Try to leave a few minutes at the end of the exam to go back and read over your answers.

Always use a Clear Writing Style

1) It's a good idea to start essay answers with a brief introduction and end with a conclusion.
2) Remember to start a new paragraph for each new point you want to discuss.
3) Try to use clear handwriting and pay attention to spelling, grammar and punctuation. In the 16-mark question, there are an extra 4 marks available for SPaG.

Plan your essay answers

1) For longer essay questions, it's important to make a quick plan before you start writing.
2) Think about what the key words are in the question. Scribble a quick plan of your main points — cross through this neatly at the end so it isn't marked.

> You don't need to plan answers for the shorter questions.

Stay Focused on the question

1) Make sure that you answer the question. Don't just chuck in everything you know about the topic.
2) You've got to be accurate — make sure you include precise details like the dates of medical discoveries and the names of people who made them.

> It might help to write the first sentence of every paragraph in a way that addresses the question, e.g. "Another reason why medicine didn't change much in the medieval period was..."

Skills for the Thematic Study

The main part of <u>Paper 1</u> is the <u>Thematic Study</u>. There are three questions which test <u>two main skills</u>.

There are Three types of exam question in the Thematic Study

1) In the first question, you'll need to <u>compare two</u> different <u>time periods</u>. You'll be asked about a <u>similarity</u> or <u>difference</u> between these two periods, and will need to explain your answer.

> Explain one way that beliefs about the spread of disease in the medieval period were similar to those in the period c.1500-c.1700.   [4 marks]

2) The next question will ask you to <u>explain</u> something about a change — e.g. <u>why</u> something changed over a certain time, or why changes were <u>slow</u> / <u>quick</u> to happen. Make sure you <u>analyse</u> each point fully, including plenty of <u>detail</u>.

> Explain why access to healthcare improved rapidly in the twentieth century.   [12 marks]

3) The final task will cover at least <u>200 years</u> of history. You'll get a choice of two questions — answer the one you're most <u>comfortable</u> with. Each one will give a <u>statement</u> and you'll be asked how <u>far you agree</u> with it.

> 'The discovery of anaesthetics was the most important development in surgery between c.1700 and c.1900.' Explain how far you agree.   [16 marks]

4) Decide your opinion <u>before</u> you begin writing, state it clearly at the start and end of your answer, and include evidence for <u>both sides</u> of the argument.

> There are also 4 marks available for spelling, punctuation, grammar and the use of specialist terminology in the final task, so it's worth 20 marks in total.

> In question types 2) and 3), you'll be given two '<u>stimulus points</u>' (hints about things you could include in your answer). You don't <u>have</u> to include them, so <u>don't panic</u> if you can't remember much about them. But you <u>must</u> always give <u>other information</u> to get full marks.

The thematic study tests Two Main Skills

Knowledge and Understanding

1) For <u>all the thematic study questions</u>, you'll get marks for showing <u>knowledge and understanding</u> of the <u>key features</u> of the topic.

2) You'll need to use <u>accurate</u> and <u>relevant</u> information to <u>explain</u> <u>changes</u> in different historical periods. You'll also need to use <u>evidence</u> to <u>support</u> your answers to the longer essay questions.

> The <u>Knowledge and Understanding</u> activities in this book will help you to revise the <u>important facts</u> for each period so that you have <u>plenty of information</u> to help you in the exam.

Thinking Historically

1) The thematic study is divided into <u>four</u> different <u>time periods</u>, but you'll need to think about the topic as a <u>whole</u> for the exam and make <u>links</u> between different periods.

2) The study focuses on what <u>changed</u> (and <u>what didn't change</u>) over time and <u>why</u>. The questions will ask you about historical concepts like <u>continuity</u>, <u>change</u>, <u>similarity</u> and <u>difference</u>. You'll also need to know the <u>main factors</u> that caused or prevented change — things like <u>religion</u>, <u>technology</u> and <u>people's attitudes</u>.

> The <u>Thinking Historically</u> activities will get you thinking about the <u>significance</u> of <u>different factors</u>, <u>turning points</u> in medicine and how much <u>change</u> or <u>continuity</u> there has been across different periods in history.

The Thematic Study is all about change over time...

The Thematic Study appears a bit daunting because it covers such a long period of time but don't worry — in this book the topic is broken down into different time periods to help you.

Skills for the Historic Environment

These two pages will help you understand the Historic Environment section of the exam. There are two main skills you'll need — a good knowledge of the Western Front and the ability to use sources.

You'll need to Write About the Key Features of the Western Front

1) In the Historic Environment section of the exam, you'll be expected to show your knowledge and understanding of medicine on the Western Front, as well as your ability to analyse sources.

2) The activities in the Historic Environment section of this book will help you to practise the skills you'll need for the exam.

Knowledge and Understanding

1) In the Historic Environment section, you'll need to be able to identify and talk about the key features of your site — in this case, the Western Front.

2) Question 1 will ask you to describe two different features of a certain aspect of the Western Front.

3) To get all four marks, you'll need to identify two features and then give a little bit of extra information that's relevant to each one.

> Key features of a historical site are any details, characteristics or unique features that stand out and make the site, or part of it, special. They are the main or most important characteristics of the site. For example, the layout and organisation of the trenches, trench conditions, illnesses and injuries caused by trench warfare, and the Chain of Evacuation are all key features of the Western Front.

Give a description of **two** features of the FANY (First Aid Nursing Yeomanry Corps).   [4 marks]

> You only need to talk about two key features — writing about more won't get you extra marks.

> Identify a feature, then add some supporting information that gives a bit more detail.

The FANY provided transport and ambulance services for the Allied armies on the Western Front. They staffed two important ambulance convoys — the Calais Convoy and the St. Omer Convoy.
     As well as transporting soldiers, the FANY also helped to keep soldiers well fed. They ran mobile soup kitchens, hospital canteens and moved rations between coastal ports and the front line.

> Make sure your supporting information is linked to the feature that you've talked about.

4) To answer Question 1, you'll need to have a good knowledge and understanding of the Western Front.

5) Having a good knowledge of medicine on the Western Front will also help you to answer both parts of Question 2, which are about analysing sources.

6) You'll need to use your knowledge to put the sources into context — use what you know to help you make judgements about each source. Don't just bring in random bits of information — make sure you stick to stuff that's relevant to the question.

> The Knowledge and Understanding activities throughout this book will help you to learn the important facts you'll need for this part of the exam.

Skills for the Historic Environment

You'll also have to Analyse two different Sources

Source Analysis

In Question 2 of the <u>Historic Environment</u> section, you'll be given <u>two sources</u>:

1) Question 2(a) will ask you to consider <u>how useful</u> the sources are for a particular investigation. The <u>investigation</u> will have a <u>specific focus</u>.

2) For each source, you should think about:
   - The <u>date</u> — when it was produced
   - The <u>author</u> — who produced it and where
   - The <u>purpose</u> — why it might have been produced
   - The <u>content</u> — what the source shows

3) In your answer, you'll need to explain how these factors affect the <u>usefulness</u> of the source.

> How useful are Sources A and B for studying the evacuation of the wounded on the Western Front? Use both sources and your own knowledge to support your answer.   [8 marks]

> You may be given both written and visual sources, but you should handle them both in the same way.

> For example, this image is <u>useful for studying</u> the problems involved in <u>evacuating the wounded</u> because it shows stretcher bearers <u>struggling to carry</u> a wounded man across shell-damaged terrain during a battle. This can help us to <u>understand the dangers and difficulties</u> that stretcher bearers faced when they were evacuating injured soldiers.

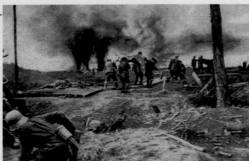

© Historical Images Archive / Alamy Stock Photo

4) Question 2(b) in the exam will ask you <u>how</u> you'd use <u>one</u> of the two sources to <u>find out more</u> about the issue in the first part of the question.

5) You'll be asked for <u>four pieces</u> of information — you'll get a mark for <u>each one</u>.

> How could you further investigate Source A to learn more about the evacuation of the wounded?   [4 marks]

---

1) First, you need to <u>identify</u> a <u>detail</u> in the source that you'd like to <u>investigate</u>. For written sources, a detail could be a short <u>extract</u> from the text. For image sources, it could be something that <u>features in the image</u>.

2) Then you need to create a <u>question</u> that will help you find out <u>a bit more information</u> about the <u>detail</u> that you've picked out. Your <u>question</u> should help you <u>follow up</u> on the <u>issue</u> that's been identified in the first part of the <u>exam question</u>.

3) After you've written your <u>question</u>, you need to say which <u>type of source</u> you could use to <u>answer</u> it. Think about what <u>kind of information</u> you need to answer your question and then identify a source that could <u>tell you</u> that information.

4) Finally, you need to <u>explain how</u> the source will help you to <u>answer</u> the question. It's a good idea to think about the <u>strengths</u> of the source and why it would be <u>useful</u> for your investigation.

> The <u>Source Analysis</u> activities in this book will help you to practise <u>understanding</u> sources, analysing their <u>usefulness</u> and using them to plan your own <u>historical investigations</u>.

EXAM TIP

Barbecue sauce has no weaknesses...

Analysing sources might seem overwhelming at first, but writing down important details such as the date, author, purpose and content of the source before you answer the question will help.

Disease and the Supernatural

Without further ado, let's dive into the content of the <u>thematic study</u> — medicine in Britain. The first section looks at medicine in the period <u>c.1250-c.1500</u> when the treatment of disease was a bit... well... <u>medieval</u>.

Disease was thought to have Supernatural Causes

1) Many people believed that disease was a <u>punishment from God</u> for people's <u>sins</u>. They thought that disease existed to show them the error of their ways and to make them become better people. Therefore, they thought that this meant the way to cure disease was through <u>prayer</u> and <u>repentance</u>.

2) Disease was also thought to be caused by evil supernatural beings, like <u>demons</u> or <u>witches</u>. Witches were believed to be behind outbreaks of disease — many people were tried as witches and executed.

3) People believed that some diseases could be caused by <u>evil spirits</u> living inside someone. Members of the Church performed <u>exorcisms</u>, using chants to remove the spirit from the person's body.

The Church had a big Influence on medieval medicine

1) The <u>Roman Catholic Church</u> was an extremely powerful organisation in medieval Europe. It dominated the way people studied and thought about a range of topics, including medicine.

2) The Church encouraged people to believe that disease was a <u>punishment from God</u>, rather than having a natural cause. This <u>prevented</u> people from trying to <u>find cures</u> for disease — if disease was a punishment from God, all you could do was pray and repent.

3) The Church made sure that scholars of medicine learned the works of <u>Galen</u> (see p.8) as his ideas fit the Christian belief that God <u>created</u> human bodies and made them to be <u>perfect</u>. Because Galen's work was so central to medical teaching, it was <u>difficult</u> to <u>disagree</u> with him.

4) The Church outlawed <u>dissection</u>. This meant that medieval doctors <u>couldn't</u> discover ideas about human <u>anatomy</u> for themselves — they instead had to learn Galen's <u>incorrect</u> ideas that were based on animal dissection.

Comment and Analysis

The Church's influence over medieval medicine meant that there was <u>very little change</u> in ideas about the cause of disease until the Renaissance — the Church and its messages were so influential that people were <u>unable to question them</u>.

Astrology was used to Diagnose disease

1) <u>Astrology</u> is the idea that the <u>movements</u> of the <u>planets</u> and <u>stars</u> have an effect on the Earth and on people. Astrologers in medieval England believed that these movements could cause <u>disease</u>.

2) Astrology was a <u>new way</u> of diagnosing disease. It was developed in <u>Arabic</u> medicine and brought to Europe between <u>1100</u> and <u>1300</u>.

3) Medieval doctors owned a type of calendar (called an <u>almanac</u>) which included information about where particular <u>planets</u> and <u>stars</u> were at any given time, and how this related to <u>patients' illnesses</u>.

4) Different <u>star signs</u> were thought to affect different parts of the body.

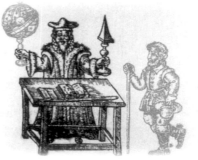

A woodcut from 1490 showing two astrologers looking at the positions of the Sun and Moon to predict the effects on people's lives.

Disease and the Supernatural

Medieval people often believed that disease had supernatural causes, such as God, witches or evil spirits. Try these activities to make sure you know the different theories about the causes of disease.

Knowledge and Understanding

1) Copy and complete the table below, explaining how medieval people dealt with the following 'causes' of disease.

Cause	How people dealt with it
a) Punishment from God	
b) Witches	
c) Evil spirits	

2) How was astrology used by doctors to diagnose disease?

Thinking Historically

1) Copy and complete the mind map below, adding points about the different ways that the Church influenced medieval medicine.

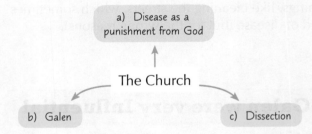

a) Disease as a punishment from God

The Church

b) Galen

c) Dissection

2) Which of the three factors mentioned above do you think was most responsible for preventing medical developments during the medieval period? Explain your answer.

3) Do you think astrology was significant in changing medieval attitudes to the causes of disease? Explain your answer.

The medieval period — a dark age for medicine...

*It's important to understand medieval people's beliefs about the causes of disease.
In the exam, you might get a question asking how these beliefs changed in later periods.*

c.1250-c.1500: Medicine in Medieval England

Rational Explanations

Some treatments in medieval England were based <u>less</u> on <u>religious faith</u> and <u>more</u> on <u>rational theories</u> and observation of the physical world. But a reason-based theory can still be <u>wrong</u>.

Medicine was dominated by the Four Humours Theory

Many medieval doctors based their <u>diagnosis</u> and <u>treatments</u> on the <u>Theory of the Four Humours</u>.

1) The Theory of the Four Humours was created by the Ancient Greek doctor <u>Hippocrates</u> (c.460-c.377 BC). Hippocrates believed that the body was made up of <u>four fluids</u> (or <u>humours</u>) — <u>blood</u>, <u>phlegm</u>, <u>yellow bile</u> and <u>black bile</u>. These were linked to the <u>four seasons</u> and the <u>four elements</u>. They needed to be in <u>balance</u> for good health.

> E.g. in <u>winter</u> we get <u>colds</u>. So Hippocrates thought that in winter the body created an excess of <u>phlegm</u>. Sadly, Hippocrates failed to see that a bunged-up nose, fevers and suchlike are <u>symptoms</u> of the disease — he thought they were the <u>cause</u>.

> E.g. someone with a <u>cold</u> (too much cold, wet <u>phlegm</u>) could be given chicken, pepper or wine (all considered <u>hot</u> and <u>dry</u>) to correct the <u>imbalance</u>.

2) The Theory of the Four Humours was developed further by another Greek doctor, <u>Galen</u>, who was born in AD 129 and worked for much of his career in <u>Rome</u>.

3) Galen believed that diseases could be treated using <u>opposites</u>. He thought that different foods, drinks, herbs and spices had a <u>humour</u>, which could <u>balance</u> the excessive humour that was causing the disease.

The Miasma Theory blamed Bad Air for causing disease

1) The <u>miasma</u> theory is the idea that <u>bad air</u> (or miasma) causes disease when someone breathes it in. This bad air may come from human <u>refuse</u>, <u>abattoirs</u> or <u>dead bodies</u> — anything that creates a <u>bad smell</u>.

2) The miasma theory originated in Ancient <u>Greece</u> and <u>Rome</u>, and was incorporated by <u>Galen</u> into the Theory of the <u>Four Humours</u>. The idea became extremely popular in medieval England.

3) The miasma theory was so influential that it lasted until the <u>1860s</u>, when it was replaced by the <u>Germ Theory</u> (see p.34). Miasma often prompted people to do <u>hygienic</u> things, like cleaning the streets, which sometimes helped to stop the spread of disease (but for the wrong reasons).

Comment and Analysis

The Four Humours and miasma were both <u>incorrect</u> theories. But they were <u>rational</u> — they assumed disease had a <u>natural</u> cause, rather than a supernatural one. This was important, as it suggested that people weren't <u>powerless</u> against disease — they could <u>investigate</u> and <u>take action</u> against it.

Hippocrates and Galen were very Influential

The work of <u>Hippocrates</u> and <u>Galen</u> was extremely influential in medical diagnosis and treatment (see p.10).

1) Hippocrates and Galen wrote down their beliefs about medicine. These were <u>translated</u> into Latin books, which were considered important texts by the <u>Roman Catholic Church</u>. Like the Bible, Hippocrates' and Galen's ideas were considered the <u>absolute truth</u>.

2) Many of their ideas were taught for <u>centuries</u> after their deaths, including the <u>incorrect</u> ones. E.g. Galen only ever dissected <u>animals</u> — animal and human bodies are very different, so some of his ideas about <u>anatomy</u> were <u>wrong</u>. Medieval doctors were <u>not allowed</u> to perform their own dissections, so they continued to learn Galen's incorrect ideas.

3) Some of Hippocrates' and Galen's ideas were so influential that they continue to be used <u>today</u>. The <u>Hippocratic Oath</u> is the <u>promise</u> made by doctors to obey rules of behaviour in their professional lives — a version of it is still in use today. Hippocrates and Galen also believed that doctors should <u>observe</u> their patients as they treat them.

Rational Explanations

These activities will help you understand rational explanations for disease during the medieval period.

Knowledge and Understanding

1) Using your own words, explain each of the headings in the boxes below.

a) Hippocrates' Theory of the Four Humours

b) How Galen developed the theory

2) Explain why a medieval doctor might have told someone with a cold to drink some wine.

3) Copy and complete the mind map below to explain what the miasma theory is.

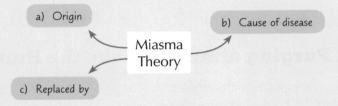

a) Origin

b) Cause of disease

Miasma Theory

c) Replaced by

4) Explain why the miasma theory sometimes helped prevent disease, even though it was incorrect.

Thinking Historically

1) Copy and complete the diagram below, explaining how each of the points below affected medieval medicine.

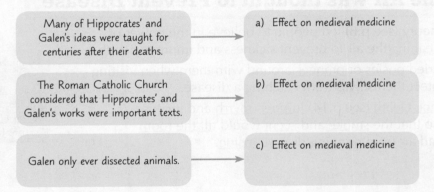

Many of Hippocrates' and Galen's ideas were taught for centuries after their deaths.

a) Effect on medieval medicine

The Roman Catholic Church considered that Hippocrates' and Galen's works were important texts.

b) Effect on medieval medicine

Galen only ever dissected animals.

c) Effect on medieval medicine

2) Do you think Hippocrates and Galen were the most important influences on medieval medicine? Explain your answer.

 The four humours — they're totally hilarious...

In the exam, it's important to take a couple of minutes before the start of longer questions to plan your answer. This will make sure that you answer the question and don't veer off topic.

Treating Disease

As the Middle Ages went on, medical treatments continued to be based on ideas we'd nowadays consider very <u>unscientific</u>. <u>Treatments</u> were <u>ambitious</u> though, and <u>theories</u> quite <u>sophisticated</u> in their <u>own ways</u>.

Prayer and Repentance were major treatments

1) Disease was believed to be a punishment from God, so sick people were encouraged to <u>pray</u>. The sick often prayed to <u>saints</u>, in the hope they would intervene and stop the illness. Medieval people also believed that <u>pilgrimages</u> to <u>holy shrines</u> (e.g. sites containing the remains of saints) could cure <u>illnesses</u>.

2) Others took their <u>repentance</u> one step further. <u>Flagellants</u> were people who whipped themselves in public in order to show God that they were sorry for their past actions. They were particularly common at times of <u>epidemics</u>, such as the Black Death (see p.14).

3) Many <u>doctors</u> had <u>superstitious beliefs</u> — e.g. some doctors used astrology to diagnose and treat illness (see p.6). Others believed that saying <u>certain words</u> when administering treatment could make that treatment more effective.

Bloodletting and Purging aimed to make the Humours balanced

1) <u>Bloodletting</u> and <u>purging</u> were popular treatments because they fitted in with the <u>Four Humours Theory</u>.

2) If someone apparently had too much blood inside them, the doctor would take some blood out of their body through <u>bloodletting</u> — they might make a small <u>cut</u> to remove the blood or use blood-sucking <u>leeches</u>.

3) Some people were accidentally <u>killed</u> because too much blood was taken.

4) <u>Purging</u> is the act of getting rid of other fluids from the body by <u>excreting</u> — doctors gave their patients <u>laxatives</u> to help the purging process.

> **Comment and Analysis**
>
> <u>Bloodletting</u> caused more deaths than it prevented, but it remained a popular treatment. This shows the strength of medieval people's <u>beliefs</u> in the face of <u>observational evidence</u>.

Purifying the Air was thought to Prevent Disease

1) The <u>miasma</u> theory (see p.8) led people to believe in the power of <u>purifying</u> or <u>cleaning</u> the air to prevent sickness and improve health.

2) Physicians carried <u>posies</u> or <u>oranges</u> around with them when visiting patients to protect themselves from catching a disease.

3) During the <u>Black Death</u> (see p.14) <u>juniper</u>, <u>myrrh</u> and <u>incense</u> were burned so that the <u>smoke</u> and <u>scent</u> would <u>fill the room</u> and prevent bad air from bringing disease <u>inside</u>.

> Purifying the air was also seen as important for helping with <u>other health conditions</u>. In the case of <u>fainting</u>, people <u>burned feathers</u> and made the patient <u>breathe in their smoke</u>.

Remedies were Early Natural Medicines

1) Remedies bought from an <u>apothecary</u>, local <u>wise woman</u> or made at <u>home</u> were all popular in medieval England and contained <u>herbs</u>, <u>spices</u>, <u>animal parts</u> and <u>minerals</u>.

2) These remedies were either <u>passed down</u> or <u>written</u> in books explaining how to mix them together. Some of these books were called '<u>Herbals</u>'.

3) Other remedies were based on <u>superstition</u>, like <u>lucky charms</u> containing '<u>powdered unicorn's horn</u>'.

Treating Disease

Now that you know all about how diseases were treated in the Middle Ages, have a go at these activities.

Knowledge and Understanding

1) Copy and complete the mind map below, adding points about the different ways that people in the medieval period treated disease.

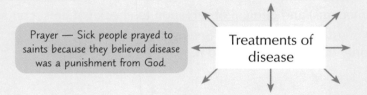

Prayer — Sick people prayed to saints because they believed disease was a punishment from God.

Treatments of disease

2) Bloodletting caused more deaths than it prevented. Why do you think medieval doctors continued to use this treatment even though it was unsafe?

Thinking Historically

1) Explain how belief in the Theory of the Four Humours and the miasma theory affected medical treatments in the medieval period.

2) Copy and complete the table below by giving a piece of evidence for and against each statement about medical treatments in the medieval period.

Statement	Evidence for	Evidence against
a) 'Religion was the biggest influence on medical treatments in the medieval period.'		
b) 'Medieval people mostly made medical treatments from things they found in the world around them.'		
c) 'Medical treatments in the medieval period usually caused more harm than good.'		

3) Explain whether, overall, you agree or disagree with each statement in the table above.

EXAM TIP

Medieval medical treatment was varied and diverse...

You might get a question in the exam on the similarities or differences between medical treatments in the medieval period and a later period — so make sure you know them well.

c.1250-c.1500: Medicine in Medieval England

Treating Disease

If you were ill in the Middle Ages, you <u>couldn't</u> just go to your <u>local GP</u>. But as there were <u>various</u> kinds of medical healers, there could still be an element of '<u>patient choice</u>'...

Physicians had little Practical Experience

1) <u>Physicians</u> were <u>male doctors</u> who had trained at <u>university</u> for at least <u>seven years</u>. They read <u>ancient texts</u> as well as writings from the <u>Islamic world</u>, but their training involved little <u>practical experience</u>.

2) Physicians used handbooks (vademecums) and <u>clinical observation</u> to check patients' conditions.

3) In 1300, there were less than 100 physicians in England. Seeing a physician was very <u>expensive</u> — only the <u>rich</u> could afford it.

Most sick people went to see an Apothecary

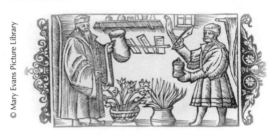

© Mary Evans Picture Library

This medieval print shows a doctor and an apothecary. The plants in the middle show the importance of herbal remedies.

1) <u>Apothecaries</u> prepared and sold <u>remedies</u> (see p.10) — and sometimes gave <u>advice</u> on how best to use them.

2) Apothecaries were trained through <u>apprenticeships</u>. Most apothecaries were men, but there were also many so-called '<u>wise women</u>', who sold <u>herbal remedies</u>.

3) Apothecaries were the most <u>common</u> form of treatment in medieval England as they were the most <u>accessible</u> for those who could not afford a physician.

> <u>Quacks</u> were people <u>without</u> any medical knowledge who sold medical treatments. They'd sell their wares at fairs and markets, and they often did more <u>harm</u> than good.

Surgery — work for Barbers, not doctors

1) Medieval surgery was very <u>dangerous</u> — there was no way to prevent <u>blood loss</u>, <u>infection</u> or <u>pain</u>. It was therefore only attempted <u>rarely</u> and for very <u>minor procedures</u>, e.g. treating hernias, pulling teeth or treating cataracts.

2) Although there were a few <u>university-trained</u>, <u>highly paid</u> surgeons, surgery as a whole was <u>not</u> a <u>respected</u> profession in medieval times — most operations were carried out by <u>barber-surgeons</u> (who also cut hair).

> **Comment and Analysis**
>
> Barber-surgeons <u>weren't</u> doctors, so they had <u>little medical training</u> or insight. This meant they had neither the ability nor the desire to experiment with new treatments.

There were Few Public Hospitals

1) There were relatively <u>few</u> hospitals in medieval Britain, so most sick people were treated at <u>home</u> by members of their <u>family</u>, mainly the <u>women</u> of the house.

2) Most <u>hospitals</u> were set up and run by <u>monasteries</u>. They were very <u>popular</u> and <u>highly regarded</u>.

3) The main purpose of hospitals was not to treat disease, but to <u>care</u> for the <u>sick</u> and <u>elderly</u>. They hospital provided its patients with <u>food</u>, <u>water</u> and a <u>warm place to stay</u>.

4) Hospitals also provided some basic medical treatments — monks also had access to <u>books</u> on healing and they <u>knew</u> how to <u>grow herbs</u> and make <u>herbal remedies</u>.

> Monastic hospitals were <u>good</u> for patients' <u>health</u> because they were more <u>hygienic</u> than elsewhere. Monasteries <u>separated</u> clean and dirty <u>water</u>. They had one water supply for <u>cooking</u> and <u>drinking</u> and one for <u>drainage</u> and <u>washing</u>, so people didn't have to drink <u>dirty water</u>. They also had <u>good systems</u> for getting rid of <u>sewage</u>.

Treating Disease

There were different kinds of healers in medieval times, but they all had their limitations. The activities on this page will help test your knowledge of each type.

Knowledge and Understanding

1) Copy and complete the table below by adding as much detail as possible about each type of healer.

Physician	Apothecary	Barber-Surgeon

2) Describe the difference between an apothecary and a quack. Why was it often dangerous to visit a quack?

3) For each person listed below, write down the type of healer or medical institution they might have visited to get treatment. Explain your answer.

   a) A poor person with a hernia

   b) A rich person with a headache

   c) A sick, elderly person with no family to support them

   d) A poor person with a cough

Thinking Historically

1) Write down a piece of evidence for and against each statement in the boxes below.

   a) 'Access to medical treatments was similar for both rich and poor people in the medieval period.'

   b) 'Hospitals in the medieval period had a big impact on helping people to get better.'

   c) 'The main reason why surgery was dangerous in the medieval period was because barber-surgeons had no training.'

2) Explain how each of the following type of healer impacted progress in treating diseases during the medieval period:

   a) Physicians

   b) Apothecaries

   c) Barber-surgeons

Anyone can be a barber-surgeon — it's not brain surgery...

Some of your marks in the exam are for using specialist terminology. Make sure you use specific terms in your exam, e.g. use 'vademecum' (if you can spell it) instead of 'handbook'.

c.1250-c.1500: Medicine in Medieval England

Case Study: The Black Death

The Black Death struck in the 14th century in Europe, and had a devastating effect. People tried to explain why it had happened, but there was little that could be done to stop the disease.

The Black Death was a devastating Epidemic

1) The Black Death was a series of plagues that first swept Europe in the mid 14th century. Two illnesses were involved:

- Bubonic plague, spread by the bites of fleas from rats carried on ships. This caused headaches and a high temperature, followed by pus-filled swellings on the skin.
- Pneumonic plague, which was airborne — it was spread by coughs and sneezes. It attacked the lungs, making it painful to breathe and causing victims to cough up blood.

2) The disease first arrived in Britain in 1348. Some historians think at least a third of the British population died as a result of the Black Death in 1348-50.

People Didn't Know what Caused the Black Death

No-one at the time knew what had caused the plague.

1) Some people believed that the Black Death was a judgement from God. They thought the cause of the disease was sin, so they tried to prevent the spread of the disease through prayer and fasting.

2) Some blamed humour imbalances, so tried to get rid of the Black Death through bloodletting and purging.

3) Those who thought that the disease was caused by miasma (see p.8) carried strong smelling herbs or lit fires to purify the air. In 1349, Edward III sent an order to the Lord Mayor of London to remove filth from the city streets, in the hope of removing bad smells.

4) Believers in astrology carried diamonds and rubies, which they believed could protect against the Black Death. People also carried charms or used 'magic' potions containing arsenic.

> **Comment and Analysis**
>
> The high death toll of the Black Death was in large part because people didn't know what caused the disease. People tried to use existing ideas about the cause of disease to come up with ways to prevent or cure the plague. But because their ideas about the cause of disease were wrong, their attempts at prevention and treatment were mostly ineffective.

Local Governments tried to Prevent the spread of the disease

1) Some people in Winchester thought that you could catch the plague from being close to the bodies of dead victims. When the town's cemetery became too full to take any more plague victims, the townspeople refused to let the bishop extend the cemetery in the town centre. Instead, they insisted that new cemeteries be built outside of the town, away from the houses.

2) The town of Gloucester tried to shut itself off from the outside world after hearing the Black Death had reached Bristol. This suggests that they thought the plague was spread by human contact. Their attempt at prevention was unsuccessful — many people in the town died of the Black Death.

3) By November 1348, the Black Death had reached London. In January 1349, King Edward III took the decision to close Parliament.

> 'Deadly pestilence had suddenly broken out in the said place and neighbourhood, and had daily increased in severity, so that grave fears were entertained for the safety of those coming here at the time.'
> King Edward III on his decision to close Parliament.

Case Study: The Black Death

Try these activities about the Black Death, people's ideas about its causes and how they tried to stop it.

Knowledge and Understanding

1) Copy and complete the table below about the two types of plague that were part of the Black Death. For each one, describe how it was spread and its main symptoms.

Type of plague	How was it spread?	Symptoms
a) Bubonic Plague		
b) Pneumonic Plague		

2) When did the Black Death arrive in Britain and what effect did it have on the population?

Thinking Historically

1) Copy and complete the mind map below by listing the different actions taken by the king, individuals and local governments and communities in response to the Black Death. Include as much detail as you can.

Responses to the Black Death

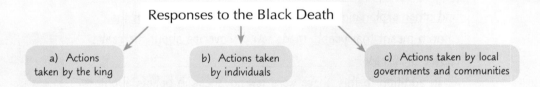

| a) Actions taken by the king | b) Actions taken by individuals | c) Actions taken by local governments and communities |

2) Explain how you think each of the following contributed to ineffective responses to the Black Death:

a) The influence of the Church

b) The lack of scientific knowledge

c) Astrology as a cause of disease

3) Why do you think medieval people were so powerless to stop the Black Death? Explain your answer.

Nobody really knew how to stop the Black Death...

Don't forget that the 14th century is referring to the 1300s. If you often get your centuries mixed up, try writing out the dates of an exam question in numbers above the words.

c.1250-c.1500: Medicine in Medieval England

Worked Exam-Style Question

The example answer below should give you some ideas about how to answer the 12-mark question.

Explain why people's understanding of the causes of disease did not advance very much in England in the medieval period.

You could mention:
- astrology
- Galen

The prompts in the question are only there as a guide. To get a high mark, you'll also need to include ideas of your own that go beyond the prompts.

You should also use your own knowledge.   [12 marks]

It's important to include factors that weren't mentioned as prompts in the question.

Giving specific examples shows you know the topic well.

This links back to the question by explaining how this factor affected the advancement of people's understanding of the causes of disease.

One reason people's understanding of the causes of disease did not advance very much in England in the medieval period was because the Roman Catholic Church encouraged the idea that disease was a punishment from God. People thought that disease existed to show them what they had done wrong and to help them become better people, so they didn't look for rational explanations for disease. The Church was very powerful and influential in medieval England so people believed its ideas and were unable or unwilling to question them. For example, when the Black Death arrived in England, many people believed the plague was a punishment from God so they didn't attempt to find other explanations for it. Therefore, the influence of the Church meant that people made few discoveries about the real causes of disease.

In addition to this, there were few advances in beliefs about the causes of disease because ancient thinkers like Galen had a strong influence on people's ideas. Galen taught that disease was caused by an imbalance of the humours, as part of the Theory of the Four Humours, and by miasma (bad air). The Church forced doctors to follow the teachings of Galen, because his ideas about the human body fit with the Church's beliefs. The Church also outlawed dissection, which prevented medieval doctors from making their own discoveries about human anatomy. Instead, they had to rely on Galen's incorrect ideas, which were based on animal dissections. The fact that the Church was so powerful meant that Galen's ideas were widely accepted so doctors and scholars were less likely to question his ideas and make discoveries about the real causes of disease.

Make sure your points are relevant to the question.

The first sentence in each paragraph links back to the question.

This is a shortened example — in the exam, you'll need to write at least one more paragraph.

Exam-Style Questions

Have a go at these exam-style questions to put everything you've learnt in this section into practice.

Exam-Style Questions

1) Explain why medical treatments remained mostly ineffective in England in the medieval period.

   You could mention:
   - trained physicians
   - quacks

   You should also use your own knowledge.   [12 marks]

2) 'The influence of the Roman Catholic Church was the main reason for the lack of change in medicine in medieval England (c.1250-c.1500).'

   Explain how far you agree with this statement.

   You could mention:
   - Galen
   - dissection

   You should also use your own knowledge.   [16 marks]

   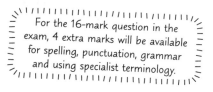
   For the 16-mark question in the exam, 4 extra marks will be available for spelling, punctuation, grammar and using specialist terminology.

3) 'Rational explanations for the causes of disease limited medical progress more than supernatural ones in medieval England (c.1250-c.1500).'

   Explain how far you agree with this statement.

   You could mention:
   - astrology
   - the Theory of the Four Humours

   You should also use your own knowledge.   [16 marks]

The Renaissance

The Renaissance was a time of <u>new ideas</u> and fresh <u>thinking</u>. People began to <u>challenge</u> old beliefs, and there were many <u>new developments</u> in doctors' <u>knowledge</u> and <u>skills</u>.

The Renaissance was a time of Continuity and Change

1) In the Renaissance there was a <u>rediscovery</u> of knowledge from classical <u>Greek</u> and <u>Roman</u> times. Western doctors gained access to the original writings of <u>Hippocrates</u>, <u>Galen</u> and <u>Avicenna</u> (a Persian physician who lived between 980 and 1037 AD). These <u>hadn't been available</u> in the medieval period. They led to <u>greater interest</u> in the <u>Four Humours</u> Theory and <u>treatment by opposites</u> (see p.8).

2) But the Renaissance also saw the emergence of <u>science</u> as we know it from the <u>magic</u> and <u>mysticism</u> of medieval medicine. People thought about how the human body worked based on <u>direct observation</u> and <u>experimentation</u>.

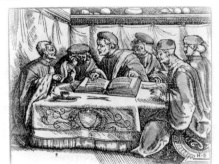

3) This was partly because many of the new books that had been found said that <u>anatomy</u> and <u>dissections</u> were very important. This encouraged people to <u>examine</u> the body themselves, and to come to their <u>own conclusions</u> about the causes of disease.

4) People began to <u>question</u> Galen's thinking and that of other ancient doctors. However, his writings <u>continued to be studied</u>.

<u>Protestant Christianity</u> spread across Europe during the <u>Reformation</u>, reducing the influence of the <u>Catholic Church</u>. Although <u>religion</u> was still <u>important</u>, the Church no longer had so much control over medical teaching.

This woodcut shows physicians debating over a medicine book.

The Medical Knowledge of doctors Improved

1) Many doctors in the Renaissance trained at the <u>College of Physicians</u>, which had been set up in <u>1518</u>. Here they read books by <u>Galen</u>, but also studied <u>recent</u> medical developments. <u>Dissections</u> — showing how the body actually worked — also became a <u>key part</u> of medical training.

2) The College of Physicians encouraged the <u>licensing</u> of doctors to stop the influence of <u>quacks</u>, who sold <u>fake medicines</u> (see p.12). Some of the college's physicians (such as <u>Harvey</u> — see p.22) made <u>important discoveries</u> about disease and the human body.

3) New <u>weapons</u> like <u>cannons</u> and <u>guns</u> were being used in <u>war</u>. This meant that doctors and surgeons had to treat injuries they <u>hadn't seen before</u>, forcing them to quickly find <u>new treatments</u>.

There were some <u>technological</u> developments too. <u>Peter Chamberlen</u> invented the <u>forceps</u> (probably at some point in the 1600s), which are still used today to help with <u>childbirth</u>.

4) <u>Explorations</u> abroad brought <u>new ingredients</u> for drugs back to Britain, including <u>guaiacum</u> — believed to cure syphilis — and <u>quinine</u>, a drug for <u>malaria</u> from the bark of the <u>Cinchona</u> tree.

5) In the <u>1530s</u>, Henry VIII closed down most of Britain's <u>monasteries</u> (this was called the '<u>dissolution of the monasteries</u>'). Since most hospitals had been set up and run by monasteries (see p.12), this also led to the <u>closure</u> of a large number of <u>hospitals</u>. The sudden <u>loss</u> of so many hospitals was <u>bad</u> for people's <u>health</u>.

6) The monastic hospitals were gradually <u>replaced</u> by some <u>free hospitals</u>, which were paid for by <u>charitable donations</u>. Unlike the monastic hospitals, which had been run by monks, these new hospitals were run by trained <u>physicians</u>, who focused more on <u>getting better</u> from <u>illness</u>.

The Renaissance

Medicine made some progress during the Renaissance, but many ideas about the causes and treatment of disease stayed the same. Try these activities to test your understanding.

Knowledge and Understanding

1) Explain one way that people's ideas about the causes of disease stayed the same between the medieval period and the Renaissance period.

2) In your own words, describe how developments in warfare led to advances in medicine in the Renaissance period.

3) Use the information on the previous page to write a definition for each of the following terms:

   a) Avicenna
   b) the College of Physicians
   c) guaiacum

   d) quinine
   e) the dissolution of the monasteries
   f) forceps

Thinking Historically

1) The mind maps below contain three major developments that took place during the Renaissance period. Copy and complete the mind maps by adding the ways in which each development affected medicine during the Renaissance period.

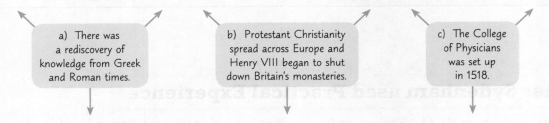

a) There was a rediscovery of knowledge from Greek and Roman times.

b) Protestant Christianity spread across Europe and Henry VIII began to shut down Britain's monasteries.

c) The College of Physicians was set up in 1518.

2) Look at the factors in the boxes below. Which one do you think was the most important cause of change in medicine during the Renaissance period? Explain your answer.

a) Institutions like the College of Physicians

b) Scientific and technological developments

c) Attitudes in society

3) Using your answer to Question 2, why do you think the other two factors were less important in causing change in medicine during the Renaissance period?

The Renaissance was an age of new ideas...

It really helps to add some important facts in your answers — a useful date, for example. But make sure they're relevant — the details should be used to support your argument.

c.1500-c.1700: The Medical Renaissance in England

Vesalius and Sydenham

Vesalius and Sydenham believed that direct observation was the best way to learn about the body. They encouraged people to gain practical experience, and to use dissection to understand anatomy.

Vesalius wrote Anatomy books with Accurate Diagrams

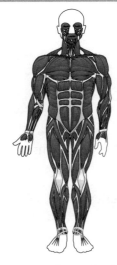

1) Vesalius was born in 1514 and was a medical professor in Padua, Italy. He believed that successful surgery would only be possible if doctors had a proper understanding of the anatomy.

2) Vesalius was able to perform dissections on criminals who had been executed. This let him study the human anatomy more closely.

3) He wrote books based on his observations using accurate diagrams to illustrate his work. The most important were 'Six Anatomical Pictures' (1538) and 'The Fabric of the Human Body' (1543).

4) His works were printed and copied (see the printing press, p.24), allowing lots of people to read about his ideas.

> Vesalius' work helped point out some of Galen's mistakes. For example, in the second edition of 'The Fabric', Vesalius showed that there were no holes in the septum of the heart.

5) Vesalius's findings encouraged others to question Galen. Doctors also realised there was more to discover about the body because of Vesalius' questioning attitude.

6) Vesalius showed that dissecting bodies was important, to find out exactly how the human body was structured. Dissection was used more and more in medical training for this reason (see p.18).

Comment and Analysis

The work of Vesalius didn't have an immediate impact on the diagnosis or treatment of disease. However, by producing a realistic description of the human anatomy and encouraging dissection, Vesalius provided an essential first step to improving them.

Thomas Sydenham used Practical Experience

1) Thomas Sydenham (1624-1689) was a Renaissance physician who worked in London. He was the son of a country squire, and fought in the English Civil War before becoming a doctor. He has been called the 'English Hippocrates' because of the big impact of his medical achievements.

2) Sydenham didn't believe in the value of theoretical knowledge. Instead he thought that it was more important to gain practical experience in treating patients. As a doctor, he made detailed observations of his patients and kept accurate records of their symptoms.

3) Sydenham thought that diseases could be classified like animals or plants — the different types of disease could be discovered using patients' symptoms.

4) Sydenham is known for showing that scarlet fever was different to measles, and for introducing laudanum to relieve pain. He was also one of the first doctors to use iron to treat anaemia, and quinine for malaria (see p.18).

5) Sydenham wrote a book called 'Medical Observations' (published in 1676), which was used as a textbook by doctors for 200 years. His descriptions of medical conditions like gout helped other doctors to diagnose their patients more easily.

Comment and Analysis

Sydenham's work on classifying diseases helped make diagnosis a more important part of doctors' work. Before, the emphasis had been on prognosis — predicting what the disease would do next.

Vesalius and Sydenham

Vesalius and Sydenham both had an impact on the development of medicine. These activities will help you to improve your understanding of their work and the discoveries they made.

Knowledge and Understanding

1) Copy and complete the table below about the work of Vesalius and Thomas Sydenham.

	Vesalius	Sydenham
a) Methods used to carry out research		
b) Important ideas and discoveries		
c) Important book(s)		
d) Influence on the future of medical training		

2) Explain the difference between diagnosis and prognosis.

Thinking Historically

1) Copy and complete the diagram below. Describe how each area of medicine changed during Vesalius' lifetime, and explain whether each change was due to the influence of Vesalius, shifting attitudes in society, technological developments or a combination of these factors.

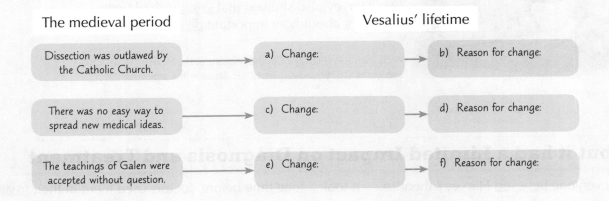

The medieval period — Vesalius' lifetime

Dissection was outlawed by the Catholic Church. → a) Change: → b) Reason for change:

There was no easy way to spread new medical ideas. → c) Change: → d) Reason for change:

The teachings of Galen were accepted without question. → e) Change: → f) Reason for change:

2) Do you think Sydenham deserves the name the 'English Hippocrates'?
Use the information on page 8 to explain your answer.

 EXAM TIP

Sydenham and Vesalius believed in direct observation...

Make sure you know how much time to spend on each question in the exam — if one question is worth twice as many marks as another, you should spend about twice as long answering it.

c.1500-c.1700: The Medical Renaissance in England

Case Study: William Harvey

<u>William Harvey</u> is a key person in the history of <u>Renaissance medicine</u>.
He made hugely important discoveries about how blood <u>circulates</u> around the body.

Harvey discovered the Circulation of the Blood

1) <u>William Harvey</u> was born in <u>1578</u> and worked in London at the <u>Royal College of Physicians</u>, before becoming <u>Royal Physician</u> to James I and Charles I.

2) Harvey studied both <u>animals</u> and <u>humans</u> for his work. He realised that he could <u>observe</u> living <u>animal</u> hearts in action, and that his findings would also apply to <u>humans</u>.

3) Before Harvey, people thought that there were <u>two kinds</u> of <u>blood</u>, and that they flowed through two <u>completely separate</u> systems of blood vessels. It was thought that:

- <u>Purple</u> 'nutrition-carrying' blood was produced in the <u>liver</u> and then flowed through <u>veins</u> to the rest of the body, where it was <u>consumed</u> (used up).
- <u>Bright red</u> 'life-giving' blood was produced in the <u>lungs</u> and flowed through <u>arteries</u> to the body, where it was also <u>consumed</u>.
- This may show the continuing influence of <u>Galen</u>, who had suggested this kind of system about 1400 years earlier.

Comment and Analysis

A new type of <u>water pump</u> was invented at around the time of Harvey's birth. This new <u>technology</u> gave Harvey a <u>comparison</u> and inspiration for how the heart worked.

4) Harvey realised this theory was <u>wrong</u>. From experiments, he knew that <u>too much</u> blood was being pumped out of the heart for it to be continually formed and consumed. Instead he thought that blood must <u>circulate</u> — it must go <u>round and round</u> the body.

Harvey's research was a Major Breakthrough in Anatomy...

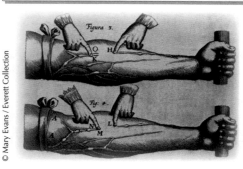

© Mary Evans / Everett Collection

1) Harvey's ideas <u>changed</u> how people understood <u>anatomy</u>. His discoveries gave doctors a new <u>map</u> showing how the <u>body</u> worked. Without this map, <u>blood transfusions</u> or <u>complex surgery</u> couldn't be attempted.

2) Harvey also showed that <u>Vesalius</u> had been <u>right</u> about how important <u>dissection</u> was.

A diagram from Harvey's 'On the Motions of the Heart and Blood' (1628), showing blood circulation in the arm.

...but it had a Limited Impact on Diagnosis and Treatment

Not everyone <u>believed</u> Harvey's theories — it took a long time before doctors used them in their <u>treatments</u>.

1) When people did attempt <u>blood transfusions</u>, they were <u>rarely successful</u> — because of blood loss, shock, and because the wrong blood types were used.

2) <u>Bloodletting</u>, which was supposed to keep the <u>Four Humours</u> in <u>balance</u> (see p.10), also continued to be performed, even though Harvey had shown the reasoning behind it to be <u>wrong</u>.

Although people knew more about the body's <u>anatomy</u> because of Harvey, <u>medical treatments</u> and <u>surgical techniques</u> were still very basic.

Case Study: William Harvey

William Harvey made some important discoveries, but not everyone accepted his findings at first. Try these activities to make sure you understand William Harvey's impact on Renaissance medicine.

Knowledge and Understanding

1) In your own words, explain what people believed about blood before William Harvey made his discoveries.

2) How did William Harvey's work change ideas about blood?

3) Explain how Harvey's work was influenced by the invention of a new type of water pump.

Thinking Historically

1) Explain how William Harvey's work developed the work of Vesalius. You can use the information on page 20 to help you.

2) In your own words, give two reasons why Harvey's theories didn't have an immediate impact on the treatment of disease.

3) Copy and complete the mind map below about William Harvey's impact on medicine in the Renaissance period.

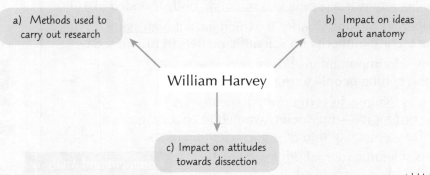

a) Methods used to carry out research

b) Impact on ideas about anatomy

William Harvey

c) Impact on attitudes towards dissection

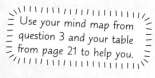
Use your mind map from question 3 and your table from page 21 to help you.

4) Do you think Vesalius, Sydenham or Harvey had the biggest effect on medical understanding in the Renaissance period? Explain your answer.

The circulation of the blood goes round and round...

Don't forget to make sure your spelling, punctuation and grammar are all accurate — there are four marks available for this in the long essay question at the end of the exam.

Transmission of Ideas

Greater scientific and medical progress in the Renaissance wasn't just the result of <u>improved understanding</u> of the <u>anatomy</u>. <u>New technology</u> allowed ideas to be circulated more easily, making change <u>even quicker</u>.

The Printing Press allowed New Ideas to be Spread

1) The <u>first British</u> printing press was set up in the <u>1470s</u>. The invention of printing accelerated the <u>rate of progress</u> in medicine (and everything else).

- Making a <u>single copy</u> of a book by <u>hand</u> could take many months or even years. Books were therefore very <u>rare</u> and <u>precious</u>.
- New ideas would have to be <u>widely accepted</u> before anyone would go to the bother of copying them by hand.
- The invention of printing allowed books to be <u>copied</u> much more <u>easily</u>.

2) <u>Students</u> in <u>universities</u> could have their own <u>textbooks</u> for the first time, letting them study in detail.

3) <u>New ideas</u> could be <u>spread</u> and <u>debated</u> more easily. <u>Ambroise Paré</u> (1510-1590) was a French army surgeon whose ideas about surgery were <u>translated</u> into different languages and <u>reprinted</u>. His works influenced <u>several other books</u> about <u>surgery</u> from this time.

4) The printing press also meant people could question <u>existing</u> ideas. At least <u>600</u> different editions of <u>Galen's</u> books were printed between 1473 and 1599. This meant that lots of people <u>knew</u> his theories. However, with so many different versions around, it was <u>unclear</u> what Galen had originally written — this made his writings seem <u>less reliable</u>.

Comment and Analysis

The <u>printing press</u> had a huge <u>impact</u> on the <u>communication</u> of ideas. Think about the impact the <u>Internet</u> has had in the last two decades — that should give you an idea of how important it was.

The Royal Society changed Perceptions of Medicine

1) The <u>Royal Society</u> was a <u>prestigious scientific body</u> founded in <u>1660</u>.

2) It was supported by King Charles II, which gave it <u>high status</u>. It's still the highest authority on scientific matters in Britain today.

3) The society was important in spreading <u>new scientific theories</u> and getting people to <u>trust new technology</u>.

4) Its motto was '<u>Nullius in verba</u>', which means '<u>take no-one's word for it</u>' — the society wanted to encourage people to be <u>sceptical</u> and to <u>question</u> scientific ideas.

5) Through its scientific journal '<u>Philosophical Transactions</u>', more people could read about new inventions and discoveries.

6) It also published Robert <u>Hooke's</u> 1665 '<u>Micrographia</u>', which showed the first drawings of a <u>flea</u> made using a <u>microscope</u>.

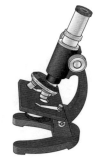

Comment and Analysis

Huge <u>progress</u> was made in the Renaissance — and the <u>printing press</u> and the <u>Royal Society</u> helped spread the <u>new ideas</u>. But because most people <u>couldn't read</u> or write, these things could only have an impact on a <u>small part</u> of society. <u>Most</u> people in the Renaissance were using the <u>same cures</u> and treatments as people in the <u>Middle Ages</u> (see p.10).

Transmission of Ideas

Use this page to help you understand the importance of the printing press and the Royal Society.

Knowledge and Understanding

1) In your own words, explain the role of the Royal Society in the Renaissance period.

2) Explain the significance of the following texts that were spread using the printing press:

   a) Ambroise Paré's books   b) 'Philosophical Transactions'   c) 'Micrographia'

3) How did the printing press encourage people to question Galen's ideas?

Thinking Historically

1) Copy and complete the mind map below to explain the effects of the printing press and the Royal Society on the way that people studied medicine.

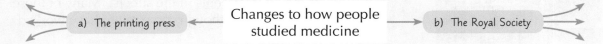

a) The printing press ← Changes to how people studied medicine → b) The Royal Society

2) 'The printing press and the Royal Society transformed society's attitudes towards medicine.'
   a) Write a paragraph agreeing with the statement above.
   b) Write a paragraph disagreeing with the statement above.
   c) Write a conclusion summarising how far you agree with the statement above.

3) The factors in the table below all had an impact on medicine during the Renaissance. Copy and complete the table by adding examples of each factor. Use information from pages 18-24.

Factor	Examples
a) **Individuals**	Vesalius
b) **Institutions**	The Royal Society
c) **Science and technology**	The printing press
d) **Attitudes in society**	

4) Which of the factors from the table above do you think was the most important for the development of medicine in the Renaissance period? Explain your answer.

The invention of printing was pretty im-press-ive...
Individuals can have an impact on the rate of change. But so can institutions, social attitudes, and developments in science and technology like the printing press. Don't forget any of these.

Medical Treatment: Continuity

Despite the rapid pace of change in the Renaissance, there was <u>continuity</u> in many aspects of medical care. For most <u>ordinary people</u>, medical treatment was <u>very similar</u> to how it had been in <u>medieval</u> times.

Some Doctors still followed Old Ideas

Many doctors were reluctant to accept that <u>Galen</u> was <u>wrong</u>. This meant that they continued to use similar treatments to the Middle Ages, like <u>bloodletting</u> and <u>purging</u> (see p.10). Doctors tended to focus more on <u>reading books</u> than on <u>treating patients</u>.

People continued to use Other Healers

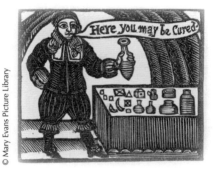

A woodcut from c.1670 showing a quack selling his 'miraculous' cures.

© Mary Evans Picture Library

1) Doctors were also still very <u>expensive</u>. As a result, most people used <u>other healers</u>, like in the <u>medieval period</u> (see p.12):

- <u>Apothecaries</u> sold medicines and drugs from their shops.
- <u>Barber-surgeons</u> were used for small operations.
- Some people turned to <u>quack doctors</u>, who sold <u>medicines</u> and <u>treatments</u> in the streets. Many of these drugs were <u>fake</u> — although some might have <u>worked</u>.

2) <u>Superstition</u> and <u>religion</u> were still important. People thought the <u>King's touch</u> could cure <u>scrofula</u> (a skin disease known as the '<u>King's Evil</u>'). <u>Thousands</u> of people with scrofula are thought to have visited King Charles I (1600-1649) in the hope of being cured.

People sought care in the Community and at Home

1) <u>Wise women</u>, who were skilled in <u>herbal remedies</u>, continued to provide medical attention within the community. This role was sometimes taken by <u>wealthy ladies</u>, who would care for <u>local families</u>.

2) People would also keep their own <u>medical</u> or <u>recipe</u> books, passed down in the family.

<u>Lady Grace Mildmay</u> (1552-1620) was a wise woman who was <u>highly educated</u> and read lots of medical books. She used her knowledge to <u>help patients</u>. She also kept <u>detailed records</u> of her treatments.

Hospitals were still Fairly Basic

1) Most Renaissance hospitals were for the <u>sick</u> and the '<u>deserving</u>' poor — those who led hardworking, respectable lives. People might have to <u>work</u> in hospital, not just be treated. Those with <u>incurable</u> or <u>infectious</u> diseases like smallpox were often not allowed in.

2) <u>St Mary of Bethlehem's</u> hospital (or '<u>Bedlam</u>') was Britain's first '<u>lunatic</u>' institution. Many of its inmates actually had <u>learning disabilities</u> or <u>epilepsy</u>, or were just <u>poor</u>. People even <u>visited</u> the hospital to watch the patients for <u>entertainment</u>.

3) Other hospitals like <u>St Bartholemew's</u> in London became centres of <u>innovation</u> and <u>new research</u>.

Comment and Analysis

<u>Hospital care</u> was still in its <u>early stages</u> in the Renaissance. Many hospitals mainly focused on <u>moral</u> or <u>spiritual</u> education. But health and sickness were becoming more of a <u>priority</u>.

c.1500-c.1700: The Medical Renaissance in England

Medical Treatment: Continuity

Lots of thing stayed the same between the medieval period and the Renaissance period. This page will help you get to grips with the aspects of medicine that didn't change much during the Renaissance.

Knowledge and Understanding

1) Give an example which shows that superstition was still important in the treatment of disease during the Renaissance period.

2) Give three examples of medical healers other than doctors who treated patients during the Renaissance period. Explain the role of each healer in Renaissance medicine.

3) Hospital care was still quite limited during this period. Copy and complete the mind map below by adding the weaknesses of hospital care during the Renaissance.

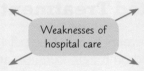

Thinking Historically

1) Copy and complete the mind map below by adding the three main reasons why you think the treatment of disease didn't change much during the Renaissance period.

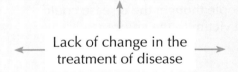

2) Copy and complete the table below by adding examples of continuity and change in medicine between the medieval period and the Renaissance period. Use information from pages 18-26 to help you. Add as many rows as you need.

Examples of continuity	Examples of change

3) Do you think there was more change or more continuity in medicine during the Renaissance period? Use your table from question 2 to help you.

Visiting a quack doctor wasn't usually very produck-tive...

It's important to understand continuity as well as change — in the exam, you could be asked to explain how a particular aspect of medicine was similar in two different periods.

Case Study: The Great Plague

The continuity of treatments was most felt when the Great Plague struck London in 1665. From prayers to bloodletting, the responses to the plague were eerily similar to the reaction to the Black Death (see p.14).

The Great Plague hit London in 1665

1) In 1665, London was struck by the Great Plague. This was a rare but deadly recurrence of the medieval Black Death.

2) London's death toll was about 100,000 — this was around 20% of the city's population.

3) Many people fled the city, but only richer people had this option.

4) Doctors and priests were often most affected because the sick went to them for help.

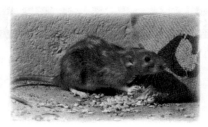

Like the Black Death, the Great Plague was spread by the bites of fleas from rats. The people at the time didn't know this, though.

Superstition still dominated Treatment

Just like responses to the Black Death 300 years before (see p.14), most treatments for the Great Plague were based on magic, religion and superstition.

1) This included wearing lucky charms or amulets, saying prayers and fasting.

2) Special remedies were made using ingredients like dried toad.

3) Bloodletting was still used, even though this probably made the plague worse — it created wounds which could become infected.

4) Other people thought that miasma caused the disease (see p.8). They carried around posies of herbs or flowers to improve the air.

5) Perhaps the most extreme treatment was strapping a live chicken to the swellings — people thought the disease could be transferred from the plague victim to the chicken.

Comment and Analysis

Living conditions were very poor in Renaissance England, so it isn't a surprise that the plague came back. Death records show that the poorest, most crowded areas of London were worst hit.

People tried to Prevent the plague from Spreading

Local councils took measures to try to stop the spread of the plague. They were largely ineffective because they didn't know the cause of the disease.

1) Councils tried to quarantine plague victims to prevent them passing on the disease to others. The victim's house was locked and a red cross was painted on their door, along with the words "Lord have mercy upon us."

2) Areas where people crowded together such as theatres were closed.

3) People tried not to touch other people. E.g. if someone had to give money in a shop, the coins might be placed in a jar of vinegar.

4) The dead bodies of plague victims were buried in mass graves away from houses. Carts organised by the authorities roamed the city to the infamous cry of "bring out your dead!", collecting corpses for burial.

5) Local councils paid for lots of cats and dogs to be killed, because they thought they carried the plague.

Comment and Analysis

The responses to the plague came from local councils — they did more to try to combat the Great Plague than they had done for the Black Death 300 years previously. But there were no national government attempts at prevention.

The plague gradually began to disappear. Many people think the Great Fire of London in 1666 helped wipe it out, by effectively sterilising large parts of London — it burned down the old, crowded houses, killing the plague bacteria.

Case Study: The Great Plague

The activities on this page will help you understand how people responded to the Great Plague.

Knowledge and Understanding

1) Why do some people think that the Great Fire of London in 1666 helped to wipe out the plague?

2) How many people died in London as a result of the Great Plague?

3) The boxes below contain three different theories about the causes of disease. Write down the responses to the Great Plague that were based on each theory.

a) The miasma theory   b) The Theory of the Four Humours   c) Punishment from God

4) In your own words, describe three ways that local councils tried to stop the Great Plague from spreading.

Thinking Historically

1) In your own words, explain why the Great Plague had such a devastating impact on the people of London. You can use the factors in the boxes below to help you write your answer.

Ideas about the cause of disease   Methods of treatment   The official response   Living conditions

2) Copy and complete the mind map below by listing the similarities between people's responses to the Black Death and the Great Plague. Use the information on page 14 to help you.

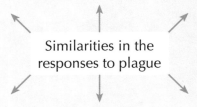

Similarities in the responses to plague

3) Why do you think that responses to the Great Plague were no more effective than responses to the Black Death? Explain your answer.

Another deadly attack of the plague...

In the exam, you might have to compare events from different periods. When you're revising, think about the similarities and differences between events like the two outbreaks of the plague.

c.1500-c.1700: The Medical Renaissance in England

Worked Exam-Style Question

The sample answer below will help you answer the four-mark question in the exam. Your answer to this question doesn't need to be long, but you need to write enough to get all four marks.

Explain one similarity between beliefs about the spread of disease in the fourteenth century and in the seventeenth century.   [4 marks]

The first sentence <u>directly</u> <u>addresses</u> the question.

This is an <u>important</u> feature of <u>both periods</u>.

One thing that was similar about people's beliefs about the spread of disease in both centuries was their belief in the miasma theory. People believed that diseases were caught by breathing in 'bad air'. They thought that bad air came from things that had a bad smell, like abattoirs or dead bodies. In the 14th century, people tried to prevent the Black Death from spreading by carrying strong smelling herbs to 'purify' the air. When the Great Plague hit London in 1665, many people carried around herbs and flowers for the same reason.

This gives more <u>specific</u> information to show an <u>understanding</u> of the miasma theory.

The answer shows a good level of knowledge by giving an example of how <u>people's actions</u> were <u>influenced</u> by their beliefs.

Exam-Style Questions

Try writing answers to the questions below to make sure you understand everything you've learnt about medicine in the Renaissance period. You'll need to use your knowledge of the medieval period too.

Exam-Style Questions

1) Explain one similarity between the methods used to prevent the spread of the Black Death in the medieval period and those used to prevent the spread of the Great Plague in the 17th century.   [4 marks]

2) Explain why ideas about the human body changed significantly in Britain during the Renaissance period (c.1500-c.1700).

   You could mention:
   • the printing press
   • the work of Vesalius

   You should also use your own knowledge.   [12 marks]

3) 'Beliefs about medicine were transformed during the Renaissance period (c.1500-c.1700).'

   Explain how far you agree with this statement.

   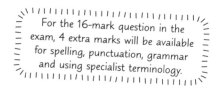
   For the 16-mark question in the exam, 4 extra marks will be available for spelling, punctuation, grammar and using specialist terminology.

   You could mention:
   • the Royal Society
   • Thomas Sydenham

   You should also use your own knowledge.   [16 marks]

Case Study: Vaccination

Until the 1700s, people had <u>few</u> effective ways to <u>prevent</u> the spread of <u>disease</u>. <u>Edward Jenner's</u> discovery of the <u>smallpox vaccine</u> was a <u>landmark</u> in the development of <u>preventive medicine</u>.

Before Jenner the only way to prevent Smallpox was Inoculation

1) In the 1700s, <u>smallpox</u> was one of the most <u>deadly</u> diseases — in 1751, over 3500 people died of smallpox in London alone.

2) At the time, the only way to prevent smallpox was through <u>inoculation</u>. This was introduced into Britain from Turkey by Lady Mary Wortley Montagu in 1718.

3) Inoculation involved making a <u>cut</u> in a patient's arm and soaking it in pus taken from the swelling of somebody who already had a <u>mild form</u> of smallpox.

> Inoculation was successful in preventing the disease, but it meant patients had to <u>experience smallpox</u> before they could become immune — some <u>died</u> as a result.

Jenner discovered a link between Smallpox and Cowpox

1) <u>Edward Jenner</u> (born in 1749) was a country doctor in <u>Gloucestershire</u>. He heard that <u>milkmaids</u> didn't get smallpox, but they did catch the much milder <u>cowpox</u>.

2) Using careful <u>scientific methods</u> Jenner investigated and discovered that it was true that people who had had <u>cowpox</u> didn't get <u>smallpox</u>.

3) In 1796 Jenner <u>tested</u> his theory. He injected a small boy, <u>James Phipps</u>, with pus from the sores of <u>Sarah Nelmes</u>, a milkmaid with cowpox. Jenner then infected him with smallpox. James <u>didn't catch</u> the disease.

4) Jenner <u>published</u> his findings in <u>1798</u>. He coined the term <u>vaccination</u> using the Latin word for cow, <u>vacca</u>.

> **Comment and Analysis**
>
> Jenner was important because he used an <u>experiment</u> to test his theory. Although experiments had been used during the Renaissance, it was still <u>unusual</u> for doctors to <u>test</u> their theories.

Jenner's vaccination was Successful despite Opposition

1) Some people <u>resisted</u> vaccination. Some <u>doctors</u> who gave the older type of inoculation saw it as a <u>threat</u> to their livelihood, and many people were <u>worried</u> about giving themselves a disease from <u>cows</u>.

2) But Jenner's discovery soon got the approval of <u>Parliament</u>, which gave Jenner <u>£10,000</u> in 1802 to open a vaccination clinic. It gave Jenner a further <u>£20,000</u> a few years later.

3) In 1840 Parliament passed an act which made vaccination against smallpox <u>free</u> for infants. In 1853 Parliament made it <u>compulsory</u>.

4) The vaccine was a <u>success</u> — it contributed to a big fall in the number of smallpox cases in Britain.

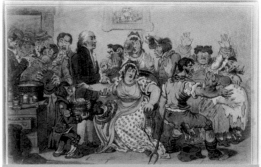

A cartoon from 1802 by James Gillray, with cows bursting out of vaccinated patients' sores. Vaccination was met with a lot of <u>opposition</u> — some groups in Britain published pamphlets against vaccination.

© Mary Evans Picture Library

> **Comment and Analysis**
>
> The government's attempts to get people vaccinated against smallpox were <u>surprising</u> given attitudes at the time. People believed in a <u>laissez-faire</u> style of government — they thought that government <u>shouldn't get involved</u> in people's lives. The vaccination policy <u>went against</u> this general attitude.

> Jenner didn't know why his vaccine worked. This <u>lack of understanding</u> meant Jenner <u>couldn't</u> develop any other vaccines. This was only possible after the Germ Theory was published (see p.34), when <u>Pasteur</u> and others worked to discover vaccines against other diseases, like chicken cholera and anthrax.

Case Study: Vaccination

Have a go at these activities to test your knowledge of the development of Jenner's smallpox vaccine.

Knowledge and Understanding

1) Explain how smallpox was prevented before Jenner developed his vaccination. Include the following key words in your explanation.

cut   inoculation   patient's arm

2) Explain why Jenner's smallpox vaccine was safer than the smallpox inoculation.

3) Copy and complete the timeline below about the decline of smallpox in Britain. Fill in all the key events between 1796 and 1853, and include as much detail as you can.

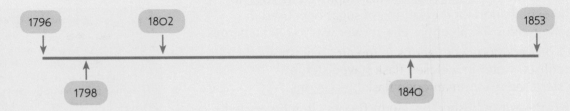

1796   1802   1853

1798   1840

4) In your own words, explain what a laissez-faire style of government is.

Thinking Historically

1) Explain why social attitudes led to some opposition to Jenner's vaccination.

2) Copy and complete the mind map below, giving examples of the role Parliament and individuals played in the development of the smallpox vaccination.

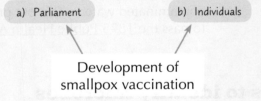

a) Parliament   b) Individuals

Development of
smallpox vaccination

3) Do you think Parliament or individuals were more important to the success of the smallpox vaccination? Explain your answer.

 EXAM TIP

Jenner's vaccine got disease prevention mooving...

Remember to use linking words and phrases like 'however', 'because of this', 'as a result' and 'therefore' to clearly show the link between an event and its causes and consequences.

c.1700-c.1900: Medicine in 18th and 19th Century Britain

The Germ Theory

Although people's understanding of anatomy had improved greatly during the Renaissance, there was still plenty to learn. The causes of disease was an area that still needed proper explanation.

People knew about Germs but hadn't linked them to Disease

1) Germs and other micro-organisms were discovered as early as the 17th century. Scientists thought that these microbes were created by decaying matter, like rotting food or human waste — this theory was known as spontaneous generation. It led people to believe that disease caused germs.

2) People still thought miasma (see p.8) was the main cause of disease. The cholera outbreak of 1831-32 (see p.42) saw the government regulate the burial of the dead bodies to stop them creating bad air.

Pasteur was the first to suggest that Germs cause disease

1) The French chemist Louis Pasteur was employed in 1857 to find the explanation for the souring of sugar beet used in fermenting industrial alcohol. His answer was to blame germs.

2) Pasteur proved there were germs in the air — he showed that sterilised water in a closed flask stayed sterile, while sterilised water in an open flask bred germs.

3) In 1861, Pasteur published his Germ Theory. In it he argued that microbes in the air caused decay, not the other way round. He also suggested that some germs caused disease.

> Pasteur's discovery was partly due to Antonie van Leeuwenhoek's invention of the microscope in the 17th century. More advanced microscopes were developed during the 1800s. They allowed scientists to see much clearer images with a lot less light distortion.

It took Time for the Germ Theory to have an Impact

1) The Germ Theory was first met with scepticism — people couldn't believe tiny microbes caused disease. It didn't help that the germ responsible for each disease had to be identified individually, as this meant it was several years before the theory became useful.

> 'I am afraid that the experiments you quote, M. Pasteur, will turn against you. The world into which you wish to take us is really too fantastic.'
> La Presse, a French Newspaper, 1860.

> 'Thanks for having, by your brilliant researches, proved to me the truth of the germ theory. You furnished me with the principle upon which alone the antiseptic system can be carried out.'
> The founder of antiseptic surgery, Joseph Lister, in a letter to Louis Pasteur, 1874.

2) The Germ Theory soon gained popularity in Britain.
- The theory inspired Joseph Lister to develop antiseptics (p.40).
- It proved John Snow's findings about cholera (p.42).
- It linked disease to poor living conditions (like squalor and contaminated water). This put pressure on the government to pass the 1875 Public Health Act (see p.44).

Robert Koch used dyes to identify microbes

1) The German scientist Robert Koch built on Pasteur's work by linking specific diseases to the particular microbe that caused them. Koch identified anthrax spores (1876) and the bacteria that cause septicaemia (1878), tuberculosis (1882) and cholera (1883).

2) Koch used revolutionary scientific methods:

- He used agar jelly to create solid cultures, allowing him to breed lots of bacteria.
- He used dyes to stain the bacteria so they were more visible under the microscope.
- He employed the newly-invented photography to record his findings.

The Germ Theory

The Germ Theory had a big impact on understanding diseases — this page will show you its significance.

Knowledge and Understanding

1) Explain the ideas behind each of the following terms:
   a) Spontaneous generation
   b) The Germ Theory

2) In your own words, explain how Pasteur proved there were germs in the air.

3) State the scientific discovery Robert Koch made in each of these years.

   a) 1876   b) 1878   c) 1882   d) 1883

4) Copy and complete the mind map below, giving examples of new technology and scientific methods which helped Robert Koch to develop his ideas on the causes of diseases.

New technology and scientific methods used by Robert Koch

Thinking Historically

1) Give one way that ideas about the causes of disease during the early 19th century were similar to ideas about the causes of disease during the Renaissance.

2) The Germ Theory and Jenner's smallpox vaccination were both important breakthroughs. Copy and complete this table, explaining why each discovery was a turning point in medicine. Use information from page 32 to help you.

Discovery	Why it was a turning point
a) The Germ Theory	
b) Smallpox vaccination	

3) Do you think the development of the Germ Theory or the smallpox vaccination had a greater effect on the prevention of disease? Explain your answer.

Pasteur's theory — more than the germ of an idea...

When you're learning about discoveries like the Germ Theory, it's important to think about how developments that came beforehand (like microscopes) made the discovery possible.

Developments in Nursing

Before the 1800s, hospitals were often <u>dirty</u> places that people associated with <u>death</u> and <u>infection</u>. <u>Florence Nightingale</u> helped change that — by improving <u>hospital hygiene</u> and raising <u>nursing standards</u>.

Florence Nightingale improved army hospitals

1) <u>Florence Nightingale</u> (1820-1910) brought a new <u>discipline</u> and <u>professionalism</u> to a job that had a very <u>bad reputation</u> at the time. Despite <u>opposition</u> from her family, she studied to become a nurse in <u>1849</u>.

2) When the <u>Crimean War</u> broke out in 1853-54, <u>horror stories</u> emerged about the <u>Barrack Hospital</u> in <u>Scutari</u>, where the British wounded were treated.

3) <u>Sidney Herbert</u>, who was both the <u>Secretary of War</u> and a friend of her family, asked for Nightingale to go to Scutari and sort out the hospital's <u>nursing care</u>.

4) The military <u>opposed</u> women nurses, as they were considered a distraction and inferior to male nurses. Nightingale went anyway, with <u>38 hand-picked nurses</u>.

5) Using methods she had learned from her training in Europe, Nightingale made sure that all the wards were <u>clean</u> and <u>hygienic</u>, that water supplies were adequate and that patients were fed properly.

6) Nightingale improved the hospital a lot. Before she arrived, the <u>death rate</u> in the hospital stood at <u>42%</u>. Two years later it had fallen to just <u>2%</u>.

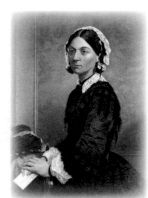

<u>Mary Seacole</u> (1805-1881) also nursed in the Crimea.

1) She learnt nursing from her mother, who ran a boarding house for soldiers in <u>Jamaica</u>.

2) In 1854, Seacole came to England to <u>volunteer</u> as a nurse in the Crimean War. She was rejected (possibly on <u>racist</u> grounds) but went anyway, paying for her <u>own</u> passage.

3) Financing herself by <u>selling goods</u> to the soldiers and travellers, she nursed soldiers on the <u>battlefields</u> and built the <u>British Hotel</u> — a small group of makeshift buildings that served as a hospital, shop and canteen for the soldiers.

4) Seacole couldn't find work as a <u>nurse</u> in England after the war and went <u>bankrupt</u> — though she did receive support due to the press interest in her story.

Nightingale used her fame to Change Nursing

1) In 1859, Nightingale published a book, '<u>Notes on Nursing</u>'. This explained her methods — it emphasised the need for hygiene and a professional attitude. It was the standard <u>textbook</u> for generations of nurses.

2) The public raised <u>£44,000</u> to help her <u>train nurses</u>, and she set up the <u>Nightingale School of Nursing</u> in <u>St. Thomas' Hospital</u>, London. Nurses were given three years of training before they could qualify. Discipline and attention to detail were important.

3) By <u>1900</u> there were <u>64,000</u> trained nurses in Britain from colleges across the country.

4) In <u>1919</u> (after Nightingale's death) the <u>Nurses Registration Act</u> was passed. This made training <u>compulsory</u> for all nurses.

> As well as improving hospital care, Florence Nightingale is credited with helping turn nursing into a <u>respectable profession</u>, particularly for <u>women</u>. This was formalised in 1916, when <u>The Royal College of Nursing</u> was founded. It began to admit <u>men</u> in 1960.

> The 1800s also saw a massive increase in <u>hospital building</u>. Hospitals became <u>cleaner</u> and <u>more specialist</u>, catering for rich patients as well as the poor.

Comment and Analysis

The Germ Theory wasn't published until 1861, so initially Florence Nightingale <u>didn't know</u> what the cause of disease was — she believed in the <u>miasma theory</u>. But her teachings suggested that good <u>hygiene</u> could prevent the spread of disease.

Developments in Nursing

Nursing changed a lot thanks to the efforts of people like Florence Nightingale and Mary Seacole. These activities will help you understand how nursing improved during the 19th century.

Knowledge and Understanding

1) In your own words, describe the events that led to Florence Nightingale becoming a nurse at the Barrack Hospital in Scutari.

2) Copy and complete the diagram, explaining what happened to Mary Seacole at different places in her life. Give as much detail as possible.

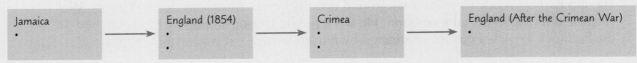

Jamaica	England (1854)	Crimea	England (After the Crimean War)

Thinking Historically

1) Explain how Florence Nightingale changed nursing in Britain. Include the following key words and date in your answer.

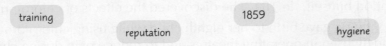

training   reputation   1859   hygiene

2) Copy and complete the table below, comparing hospitals in medieval England (p.12) and hospitals in the 19th century. Some information has already been added.

Aspect of hospital	Medieval hospitals	Hospitals in 19th century
a) **Number of hospitals**		
b) **Who ran them?**		Local authorities and volunteers
c) **Their purpose**		To treat the sick
d) **Cleanliness**		

3) How similar were hospitals in these two time periods? Use the table above to explain your answer.

4) Why do you think the Germ Theory had a limited impact on Florence Nightingale? Explain your answer.

EXAM TIP

Don't Crimea river — just learn the stuff on this page...

As well as learning and understanding the key achievements of individuals like Florence Nightingale, you also need to be able to explain why their work was significant.

c.1700-c.1900: Medicine in 18th and 19th Century Britain

Anaesthetics

Improving the hygiene and sanitation of hospitals helped to prevent many unnecessary deaths. But the two problems of pain and infection were yet to be solved. The answer to the first of those was anaesthetics.

Anaesthetics solved the problem of Pain

Pain was a problem for surgeons, especially because their patients could die from the trauma of extreme pain. Natural drugs like alcohol, opium and mandrake had long been used, but effective anaesthetics that didn't make the patient very ill were more difficult to produce.

- Nitrous oxide (laughing gas) was identified as a possible anaesthetic by British chemist Humphry Davy in 1799 — but he was ignored by surgeons at the time.
- The gas had been dismissed as a fairground novelty before American dentist Horace Wells suggested its use in his area of work. He did a public demonstration in 1845, but had the bad luck to pick a patient unaffected by nitrous oxide — it was again ignored.

- In 1842, American doctor Crawford Long discovered the anaesthetic qualities of ether, but didn't publish his work. The first public demonstration of ether as an anaesthetic was carried out in 1846 by American dental surgeon William Morton.
- Ether is an irritant and is also fairly explosive, so using it in this way was risky.

- James Simpson was a Professor of Midwifery at Edinburgh University. Looking for a safe alternative to ether that women could take during childbirth, he began to experiment on himself. In 1847, he discovered the effects of chloroform.
- After Queen Victoria gave birth to her eighth child while using chloroform in 1853, it became widely used in operating theatres and to reduce pain during childbirth.
- Chloroform sometimes affected the heart, causing patients to die suddenly.

General anaesthesia (complete unconsciousness) is risky, so local anaesthesia (numbing of the part being treated) is better for many operations. In 1884, William Halsted investigated the use of cocaine as a local anaesthetic. His self-experimentation led to a severe cocaine addiction.

Early Anaesthetics actually led to a Rise in death rates

1) Anaesthetics led to longer and more complex operations. This was because surgeons found that unconscious patients were easier to operate on, meaning they could take longer over their work.

2) Longer operating times led to higher death rates from infection, because surgeons didn't know that poor hygiene spread disease. Surgeons used very unhygienic methods.

- Surgeons didn't know that having clean clothes could save lives. Often they wore the same coats for years, which were covered in dried blood and pus from previous operations.
- Operations were often carried out in unhygienic conditions, including at the patient's house.
- Operating instruments also caused infections because they were usually unwashed and dirty.

Comment and Analysis

Anaesthetics helped solve the problem of pain, but patients were still dying from infection. This meant the attempts at more complicated surgery actually led to increased death rates amongst patients. The period between 1846 and 1870 is sometimes known as the 'Black Period' of surgery for this reason.

Anaesthetics

There are a lot of names and dates linked to the development of anaesthetics in Britain in the 1800s. To make sure all that information has sunk in, have a go at the activities on this page.

Knowledge and Understanding

1) Why are anaesthetics important during surgery?

2) Make a flashcard for each person below. Put their name on one side and describe their role in the development of anaesthetics on the other.

   a) James Simpson
   b) Humphry Davy
   c) Crawford Long
   d) Horace Wells
   e) William Halsted
   f) William Morton

3) In your own words, explain the drawbacks of each of these anaesthetics:
   a) Nitrous Oxide (laughing gas)
   b) Ether
   c) Chloroform
   d) Cocaine

4) Why is the period between 1846 and 1870 known as the 'Black Period' of surgery?

Thinking Historically

1) Which individual do you think made the most important contribution to the development of anaesthetics? Explain your answer.

2) How did developments in anaesthetics affect surgery in the short term? Give one positive effect and one negative effect.

3) Copy and complete the table below, explaining whether there was change or continuity in these aspects of surgery between the 1800s and the 1860s.

Aspect of surgery	Change or continuity?	Explanation for choice
a) Clothes worn by surgeons		
b) Use of anaesthetics		
c) Location of surgery		
d) Length of operations		

Anaesthetics revision — don't let it put you to sleep...

In the exam, remember to be specific about the information you use. For instance, rather than writing about anaesthetics in general, try to use specific examples to explain your answer.

Antiseptics

Anaesthetics had solved the problem of <u>pain</u>, but surgeons were still faced with a high death rate from operations due to the amount of <u>infection</u>. <u>Antiseptics</u> and later <u>asepsis</u> helped prevent this by killing germs.

Antisepsis and Asepsis reduce infection

There are two main approaches to <u>reducing infection</u> during an operation:

- <u>Antiseptic</u> methods are used to <u>kill germs</u> that get near surgical wounds.
- <u>Aseptic</u> surgical methods aim to <u>stop any germs</u> getting near the wound.

Joseph Lister pioneered the use of Antiseptics

1) <u>Ignaz Semmelweis</u> showed that doctors could reduce the spread of infection by washing their hands with <u>chloride of lime</u> solution between patients. However, it was very <u>unpleasant</u>, so wasn't widely used.

2) <u>Joseph Lister</u> had seen <u>carbolic acid</u> sprays used in <u>sewage works</u> to keep down the smell. He tried this in the operating theatre in the early 1860s and saw reduced infection rates.

3) Lister heard about the <u>Germ Theory</u> in 1865 — he realised that germs could be in the air, on surgical instruments and on people's hands. He started using carbolic acid on <u>instruments</u> and <u>bandages</u>.

4) The use of <u>antiseptics</u> immediately <u>reduced death rates</u> from as high as 50% in 1864-66 to around 15% in 1867-70.

5) Antiseptics allowed surgeons to operate with less fear of patients dying from infection. The <u>number of operations</u> increased tenfold between 1867 and 1912 as a result.

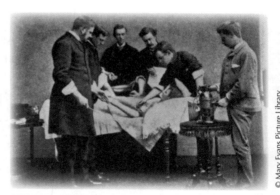

© Mary Evans Picture Library

A photograph of a surgical operation taken in the late 1800s. You can see Lister's <u>carbolic spray</u> on the table on the right. The operating theatre <u>isn't aseptic</u> though — the surgeons aren't wearing sterile gowns or surgical gloves.

Comment and Analysis

Antiseptics (and later asepsis) solved the problem of <u>infection</u>. This, combined with the use of <u>anaesthetics</u> (see p.38) to stop pain, improved British surgery — many deaths were prevented as a result of antiseptics and anaesthetics.

Asepsis reduced the need for Nasty Chemicals

Since the late 1800s, surgeons have changed their approach from <u>killing germs</u> to making a <u>germ-free</u> (aseptic) environment.

1) Instruments are carefully <u>sterilised</u> before use, usually with high temperature steam (<u>120 °C</u>).

2) Theatre staff <u>sterilise their hands</u> before entering — and wear sterile gowns, masks, gloves and hats. Surgical <u>gloves</u> were invented by <u>William Halsted</u> in <u>1889</u>.

3) The theatres themselves are kept <u>scrupulously clean</u> and fed with <u>sterile air</u>. Special tents can be placed around the operating table to maintain an area of even stricter hygiene in <u>high risk</u> cases.

4) Aseptic surgery <u>reduced</u> the need for a carbolic spray, which is <u>unpleasant</u> to get on your skin or breathe in — many doctors and nurses didn't like to use it.

Antiseptics

The introduction of antiseptics and asepsis prevented infections and greatly improved British surgery. Try out the activities below to make sure you understand the effect of these developments.

Knowledge and Understanding

1) In your own words, describe the difference between antiseptic and aseptic surgical methods.

2) How did Ignaz Semmelweis contribute to the development of antiseptics?

3) Explain how Joseph Lister's work links to the following things:

   a) sewage works

   b) the Germ Theory

4) What was the main drawback of using carbolic acid during surgery?

5) Give three ways that surgeons have created an aseptic environment since the late 1800s.

6) Copy and complete the timeline below about developments in antiseptics in the 19th century. Use information from p.38 and p.40 to fill in all the key events.

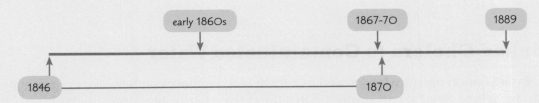

Thinking Historically

1) How did Joseph Lister change attitudes towards surgery in the 19th century?

2) Complete the mind map below, explaining the effect that antiseptics had on surgery in the 19th century. Give as much detail as possible.

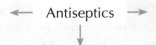

3) Using your mind map above, explain whether you think antiseptics or anaesthetics had a greater effect on 19th-century surgery.

Make a Lister them facts — then germ up on them...

You need to be confident about how surgery changed over time. Surgeons started by killing germs with antiseptic methods, and then began to stop germs using aseptic methods as well.

c.1700-c.1900: Medicine in 18th and 19th Century Britain

Case Study: Cholera in London

The industrial revolution began in the 18th century. Lots of people moved into cities like London to work in the factories. The places they lived were cramped, dirty and great for spreading diseases like cholera.

Towns had no proper Water or Waste facilities

1) Before the Germ Theory was published, people didn't understand the need for clean water or good sewerage systems. Most houses had no bathroom — they instead shared an outside toilet, called a privy.

2) Each privy was built above a cesspit. Cesspit and household waste was collected by nightmen, who threw the waste into rivers or piled it up for the rain to wash away.

3) Water companies set up water pumps in the streets, which were shared between many houses. The pump's water supply was often contaminated by waste from the cesspits or rivers.

Cholera epidemics Killed Thousands of people

1) Cholera reached Britain in 1831. By 1832, it was an epidemic — over 21,000 people in Britain died of cholera that year. The epidemics recurred in 1848, 1853-54 and 1865-66.

2) Cholera spreads when infected sewage gets into drinking water. It causes extreme diarrhoea — sufferers often die from loss of water and minerals. Both rich and poor people caught the disease.

3) At the time people didn't know what caused cholera — the best theory was miasma (see p.8). The government started regulating the burial of the dead, but this did little to halt the spread of cholera.

Snow linked Cholera to Contaminated Water

John Snow was a London doctor who showed that there was a connection between contaminated water and cholera. For a long time he had suspected that the disease was waterborne, but had very little proof.

1) When cholera broke out in the Broad Street area of London in 1854, Snow set out to test his theory. He interviewed people living in Broad Street and made a map of the area showing where cases of the disease had been. This is some of the information he collected, published in 1855 in his report 'On the Mode of Communication of Cholera':

'There were only ten deaths in houses situated decidedly nearer to another street pump. In five of these cases the families of the deceased persons informed me that they always sent to the pump in Broad Street, as they preferred the water.'	'There is a Brewery in Broad Street, near to the pump, and on perceiving that no brewer's men were registered as having died of cholera, I called on Mr. Huggins, the proprietor... He is quite certain that the workmen never obtained water from the pump in the street. There is a deep well in the brewery.'	'[A cholera victim in the West End] had not been in... Broad Street for many months. A cart went from Broad Street to West End every day, and it was the custom to take out a large bottle of the water from the pump in Broad Street, as she preferred it.'

2) Snow's investigations showed that all victims used the same water pump on Broad Street. He convinced the local council to remove the handle from the pump. This brought the cholera outbreak to an end.

3) It was later discovered that a nearby cesspit had a split lining — its waste had leaked into the pump's water supply.

Comment and Analysis

Snow's findings took a while to make an impact — it was not until the Germ Theory was published that his theory became widely accepted. But eventually Snow's findings helped lead to a change in attitudes — people realised that waterborne diseases like cholera needed a government response in order to clean up the streets and waterways. This contributed to the 1875 Public Health Act. Like Jenner (see p.32), Snow was also important for using observation and evidence to support his theory.

Case Study: Cholera in London

John Snow's discovery about cholera led to greater understanding about the importance of clean water and a properly maintained sewerage system. Try these activities to make sure you know all the important details.

Knowledge and Understanding

1) Explain what cholera is and the effect it had on people in Britain during the 19th century.

2) Using the keywords below, explain how John Snow linked cholera to contaminated water.

> Broad Street   waterborne   water pump handle

3) Copy and complete the table below, giving details about John Snow's work on cholera and Edward Jenner's work on the smallpox vaccination.

Work on disease	John Snow	Edward Jenner
a) How they tested their theory		
b) How ideas were spread		
c) Reaction from authorities		

Thinking Historically

1) Copy and complete the mind map, explaining how the following social factors contributed to the spread of cholera.

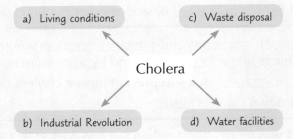

a) Living conditions   c) Waste disposal

Cholera

b) Industrial Revolution   d) Water facilities

2) How did the work of John Snow help to change attitudes to public health in the late 1800s?

If anyone knows the cause of cholera, John Snows...

When you're explaining how far you agree with a statement, you can't ignore opinions that don't match your own. You'll lose marks if you don't talk about both sides of the argument.

c.1700-c.1900: Medicine in 18th and 19th Century Britain

The Public Health Act, 1875

Before 1875, there was <u>little effort</u> to improve public health — people <u>didn't know</u> what caused disease, and they believed the government shouldn't do anything about it. The <u>Public Health Act</u> of <u>1875</u> changed this.

Earlier attempts to improve Public Health had Limited Success

1) In 1842, <u>Edwin Chadwick</u> published a report suggesting that <u>poor living conditions</u> caused <u>poor health</u>.

2) Chadwick's report led to the <u>1848 Public Health Act</u>. The Act set up a central <u>Board of Health</u> and let local councils set up their own boards of health.

3) In 1858, sewage in the River Thames made a '<u>Great Stink</u>' in the middle of London. This forced the government to plan a <u>new sewer system</u>, which opened in 1865.

> The 1848 Act's impact was <u>limited</u> — towns <u>could</u> set up health boards but very <u>few chose to</u>, and those that did often <u>refused</u> to spend any money.

Public Opinion began to Change

For most of the 19th century, people believed in a <u>laissez-faire</u> style of government — they thought the government <u>shouldn't intervene</u> in public health. But then things began to <u>change</u>.

1) <u>Snow's</u> discovery of the link between dirty water and cholera (see p.42) and Pasteur's <u>Germ Theory</u> (see p.34) showed that cleaning up towns could stop the spread of disease.

2) In 1867, the <u>Second Reform Act</u> was passed. It gave an additional <u>1 million men</u> the vote, most of whom were industrial <u>workers</u>.

3) Writers like <u>Charles Dickens</u> and philanthropists like <u>Octavia Hill</u> helped <u>change attitudes</u> towards the poor, who suffered the worst conditions.

Comment and Analysis

Now that they had the vote, <u>workers</u> could put <u>pressure</u> on the government to listen to concerns about health. For the first time, politicians had to address <u>workers' concerns</u> in order to <u>stay in power</u>.

The 1875 Act improved Public Health

In the 1870s, the government finally took action to <u>improve public health</u>.

1) In 1871-72, the government followed the Royal Sanitary Commission's proposal to form the <u>Local Government Board</u> and divide Britain into '<u>sanitary areas</u>' administered by officers for public health.

2) In 1875, the government of <u>Benjamin Disraeli</u> passed another <u>Public Health Act</u>. It forced councils to:

- Appoint <u>health inspectors</u> and <u>sanitary inspectors</u> who made sure that laws on things like <u>water supplies</u> and <u>hygiene</u> were being <u>followed</u>.
- Maintain <u>sewerage systems</u> to prevent further cholera outbreaks.
- Keep their town's <u>streets clean</u>.

3) The 1875 Public Health Act was <u>more effective</u> than the one passed in 1848 because it was <u>compulsory</u>.

4) In 1875, Disraeli also brought in the <u>Artisans' Dwellings Act</u>, which let local councils <u>buy slums</u> with poor living conditions and <u>rebuild them</u> in a way that fit new government-backed housing standards.

5) Other important reforms included the 1876 <u>River Pollution Prevention Act</u>, which stopped people from dumping sewage or industrial waste into rivers.

Comment and Analysis

Just as the government used the work of Jenner to make vaccination compulsory (see p.32), the 1875 Act built on the work of several individuals, including <u>John Snow</u> and <u>Louis Pasteur</u>. The <u>scientific proof</u> these individuals provided, combined with a <u>change in attitudes</u> towards the role of government, helped put pressure on the government to act.

The Public Health Act, 1875

SKILLS PRACTICE

The Public Health Act of 1875 did a lot to improve sanitation in towns and cities. Try these activities to check you understand what the government did to help make Britain a cleaner place.

Knowledge and Understanding

1) In your own words, describe how Edwin Chadwick contributed to improvements in public health.

2) Explain why the 1875 Public Health Act was more successful than the 1848 Public Health Act.

3) Explain how each of the following acts made Britain a healthier place to live.

   a) 1875 Public Health Act   b) 1875 Artisans' Dwellings Act   c) 1876 River Pollution Prevention Act

Thinking Historically

1) Copy and complete the mind map, explaining why attitudes towards the government's involvement in healthcare changed during the 19th century. Use ideas from the whole of this section.

Snow's discovery — showed the need for a government response to prevent the spread of diseases like cholera.

← Reasons for changing attitudes to government involvement in healthcare →

2) 'The government was the most significant factor in improving the prevention of disease between c.1700 and c.1900.' Use the table to help you structure each paragraph of an essay explaining how far you agree with this view.

Point	Evidence	Why evidence supports point?
The government improved the prevention of disease by forcing councils to address the issue of public sanitation.	The 1875 Public Health Act made councils appoint health inspectors who enforced laws about water supplies and hygiene.	Cholera was proven to be a waterborne disease, so the government's increased efforts to improve public sanitation and water supplies was significant in preventing further outbreaks.

Add three rows to the table to plan three more paragraphs.

Make sure you include arguments for and against the statement.

Talk about other important factors from this time period too.

EXAM TIP

Turns out laissez-faire had made things less fair...

There may be many reasons why a historical event happened, e.g. the government taking action to prevent disease. Try to only use the strongest, most relevant examples to back up your point.

c.1700-c.1900: Medicine in 18th and 19th Century Britain

Exam-Style Questions

Now test your knowledge on medicine in 18th and 19th century Britain by answering these exam-style questions. You'll need to use information that you've learnt about medieval and Renaissance medicine too.

Exam-Style Questions

1) Explain one difference between ideas about the prevention of disease in the Renaissance (c.1500-c.1700) and the period c.1700-c.1900. [4 marks]

2) Explain why there were improvements in surgery during the 19th century.

   You could mention:
   - the work of Joseph Lister
   - the development of anaesthetics

   You should also use your own knowledge. [12 marks]

3) 'The role of individuals was the most important factor in the development of health and medicine in Britain between c.1500 and c.1900.'

   Explain how far you agree with this statement.

   You could mention:
   - the work of John Snow
   - the role of the government

   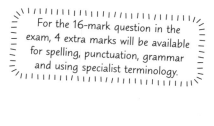
   For the 16-mark question in the exam, 4 extra marks will be available for spelling, punctuation, grammar and using specialist terminology.

   You should also use your own knowledge. [16 marks]

Exam-Style Questions

Exam-Style Questions

4) Explain one difference between ideas about the causes of disease
in the medieval period (c.1250-c.1500) and the period c.1700-c.1900.   [4 marks]

5) Explain why the prevention of disease improved rapidly during the 19th century.

    You could mention:
    * the 1875 Public Health Act
    * developments in nursing

    You should also use your own knowledge.   [12 marks]

6) 'Pasteur's Germ Theory was an important breakthrough in
the improvement of people's health in 19th century Britain.'

    Explain how far you agree with this statement.

    You could mention:
    * miasma theory
    * the work of Robert Koch

    You should also use your own knowledge.   [16 marks]

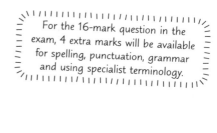

For the 16-mark question in the exam, 4 extra marks will be available for spelling, punctuation, grammar and using specialist terminology.

Modern Ideas on the Causes of Disease

The Germ Theory (see p.34) was a major breakthrough in identifying the causes of disease, but identifying bacteria couldn't explain every disease. Viruses, genetics and lifestyle were all found to impact on health.

Viruses were discovered at the turn of the century

Despite their successes with bacteria, Pasteur and Koch (see p.34) were unable to find the cause of some diseases, as they were caused by microbes called viruses, which were too small to see under a microscope.

1) In 1892 the Russian microbiologist Dmitry Ivanovsky investigated mosaic, a disease that was killing tobacco plants. He found that the cause was an extremely small microbe that remained in water even after bacteria were removed. In 1898, the Dutch scientist Martinus Beijernick found that these microbes had different properties to bacteria — he labelled these microbes viruses.

2) The discovery of viruses led to their successful treatment. Unlike bacteria, viruses aren't destroyed by antibiotics (see p.52). Instead, doctors can prescribe antiviral drugs, but they only prevent a viral infection from growing — only the body's immune system can destroy a virus for good.

DNA has given an insight into Genetic Conditions

1) Genes are the chemical 'instructions' that plan out human characteristics, like sex and hair colour. They are stored in cells as DNA. Your DNA is a mix of your parents' DNA.

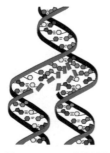

The structure of DNA is a double helix.

2) The structure of DNA, a double helix (a kind of spiral) that can reproduce itself by splitting, was first described in 1953 by Francis Crick and James Watson.

3) Watson and Crick's discovery allowed other scientists to find the genes that cause genetic conditions — diseases that are passed on from one generation to another. These include cystic fibrosis, haemophilia and sickle-cell anaemia.

4) Knowledge of genetic conditions has improved diagnosis and treatment of them. Scientists can now produce a synthetic protein to replicate the work of a faulty gene and treat inherited conditions using techniques like gene therapy.

One of the biggest breakthroughs in genetic research was made in 2003 with the completion of the Human Genome Project — this identified all the genes in human DNA.

Lifestyle Factors can increase the Risk of some Diseases

A healthy diet, exercise and other lifestyle factors have long been suggested as ways to prevent illness, but it was only in the 20th century that lifestyle choices were linked to particular health conditions:

1) Smoking has been shown to cause lung cancer (see p.62).
2) Obesity increases the chance of getting heart disease or diabetes.
3) Drinking too much alcohol has been shown to cause liver disease.
4) Overexposure to ultraviolet radiation (e.g. from sunlight) can cause skin cancer.

Comment and Analysis

The advances in science and technology since 1900 have shown that there is not just one cause of disease. In addition to bacteria, we now know that disease can be caused by viral infections, genetic mutations and our lifestyle choices. This makes their treatment and prevention even more complex — with so many different causes, treatment needs to be more targeted to the specific disease.

Modern Ideas on the Causes of Disease

This section covers more recent developments in medicine — some of which are still used today. Start off with these activities to make sure you understand the significance of viruses, DNA and lifestyle factors.

Knowledge and Understanding

1) In your own words, explain how the following individuals contributed to understanding about the causes of disease.
   a) Dmitry Ivanovsky
   b) Martinus Beijernick
   c) Francis Crick and James Watson

2) What is meant by the term 'genetic condition'? Give two examples of genetic conditions.

3) Copy and complete the mind map below about the lifestyle factors that can negatively affect a person's health. Give examples of diseases which are linked to each lifestyle factor.

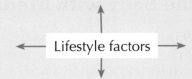

Thinking Historically

1) Do you think the discovery of viruses or the discovery of DNA had a bigger impact on modern medicine? Give a reason for your answer.

2) Copy and complete the table below, listing ideas about the different causes of disease in each time period.

Renaissance England (c.1500-c.1700)	c.1900-Present

3) Using the table above, explain whether ideas about the causes of disease were similar or different between these two time periods and suggest why you think this was.

Watson and Crick described DNA — they're gene-iuses...

Just because a concept or topic is modern, it doesn't mean you should assume the examiner knows what you're talking about. You still need to back up your points with solid examples.

Developments in Diagnosis

New causes of disease demanded new ways of diagnosing them. These new methods were introduced rapidly in the 20th century, due to innovations in science and technology, from computers to X-rays.

Blood Tests allow doctors to Diagnose more illnesses

Blood tests were first introduced to test blood groups before blood transfusions (see p.56). Since then, blood tests have been used to test for a range of diseases.

1) Blood tests can be used to check a patient's cholesterol level. This can help diagnose their chance of suffering a heart attack or stroke.

2) Blood tests can be used to check a patient's DNA (see p.48). This can help diagnose a genetic condition, like haemophilia or cystic fibrosis.

3) Some blood tests can be used to show whether a patient has a certain type of cancer, including ovarian cancer, prostate cancer and breast cancer.

> Blood tests make diagnosis more accurate, providing doctors with clearer information of what is wrong. This means they can be more confident when deciding how best to treat their patients.

Doctors can see more of the body with Medical Scans

1) The use of medical scans began in 1895 when Wilhelm Röntgen discovered X-rays. They pass easily through soft flesh, but less well through bone. They also affect photographic film. These factors allowed simple X-ray images to be produced by directing X-rays at a body part in front of a photographic plate.

2) Advances in computers allowed doctors to use ultrasound scanning — this uses high frequency sound waves, which bounce off the patient's organs and other tissues to create an image of them on the computer.

3) Computed Tomography (CT or CAT) scans were invented in 1972 by Godfrey Hounsfield. They use X-rays and a computer to make detailed images of parts of the patient's body.

4) Magnetic Resonance Imaging (MRI) scans were initially invented in 1970s but became widely used in the 1980s. These use extremely powerful radio waves and magnetic fields to construct images.

© Photo Researchers / Mary Evans Picture Library

An X-ray image of a hand from 1904. Early medical scans used dyes so that blood vessels and organs showed up on the X-ray images. These were swallowed or injected into the patient.

Comment and Analysis

Improvements in technology, like medical scans, have given doctors a much more detailed picture of what's going on inside their patient's body. This has enabled them to intervene much earlier, before the disease has become too advanced. Early treatment is generally more effective and has a higher chance of success.

Patients can now Monitor their own bodies

Since around 1900, devices have been introduced to allow doctors and patients to monitor the body.

1) Blood pressure monitors were invented and developed in the 1880s and 1890s. They let doctors and patients see whether disease, lifestyle factors or medicines are causing high blood pressure, which can cause damage to the heart.

2) Blood sugar monitors were introduced in the mid-20th century. They allow those with diabetes to make sure their blood sugar is at the right level.

> An important change in the 20th century is the use of monitoring devices by people in their own homes — this has allowed individuals greater control over their own health.

Developments in Diagnosis

The developments came thick and fast between 1895 and the late 20th century. Complete the activities below to help you understand what led to these advancements and the impact they have on doctors today.

Knowledge and Understanding

1) Copy and complete the timeline below by filling in the developments in diagnosis that happened between the late 1800s and late 1900s.

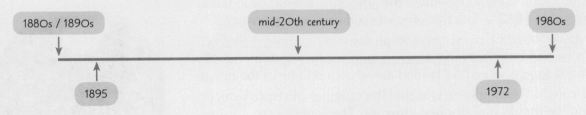

| 1880s / 1890s | mid-20th century | 1980s |

1895   1972

2) Using the keywords below, explain what ultrasound scanning is.

high frequency   organs   computer

Thinking Historically

1) In your own words, explain the effect that each of these scientific developments has had on medicine.

a) Blood tests   b) X-rays   c) Blood pressure monitors

2) Which of the three developments listed above do you think has had the most significant effect on modern medicine? Explain your answer.

3) Explain how similar the methods of diagnosis were between the medieval period and c.1900-present.

4) 'Scientific discoveries were more important than new technology to the development of medicine in the 20th century.'
a) Write a paragraph agreeing with the statement above.
b) Write a paragraph disagreeing with the statement above.
c) Write a paragraph summarising how far you agree with the statement above.

You can use details from pages 48 and 50 to help you.

EXAM TIP

I've taken an X-ray of my pet — I call it a cat scan...

In the exam, you only have a limited amount of time to answer each question. If you're spending too long on one question, finish your point then move on to the next question.

Case Study: Penicillin

In the 1800s, Pasteur discovered that <u>bacteria</u> cause disease. But it wasn't until the 1900s that doctors were able to <u>treat</u> bacterial diseases. This was partly due to the discovery of <u>penicillin</u>, the first <u>antibiotic</u>.

Fleming discovered Penicillin — the first Antibiotic

1) <u>Alexander Fleming</u> saw many soldiers die of septic wounds caused by <u>staphylococcal</u> bacteria when he was working in an army hospital during the <u>First World War</u>.

2) Searching for a cure he identified the <u>antiseptic</u> substance in tears, <u>lysozyme</u>, in 1922 — but this only worked on <u>some</u> germs.

3) One day in 1928 he came to clean up some old <u>culture dishes</u> on which he had been growing <u>staphylococci</u> for his experiments. By chance, a <u>fungal spore</u> had landed and grown on one of the dishes.

4) What caught Fleming's eye was that the <u>colonies</u> of staphylococci around the <u>mould</u> had stopped growing. The <u>fungus</u> was identified as <u>Penicillium notatum</u>. It produced a substance that <u>killed</u> bacteria. This substance was given the name <u>penicillin</u>.

5) Fleming <u>published</u> his findings in articles between 1929 and 1931. However, <u>nobody</u> was willing to <u>fund</u> further research, so he was <u>unable</u> to take his work further. The industrial production of penicillin still needed to be developed.

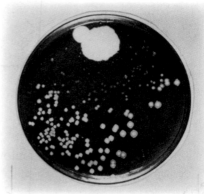

© Mary Evans Picture Library

The original plate on which Fleming first observed the growth of Penicillium notatum.

Florey and Chain found a way to Purify Penicillin

1) Since it is a natural product, penicillin needs to be <u>purified</u>. A breakthrough was made by <u>Howard Florey's</u> team in Oxford between 1938 and 1940. <u>Ernst Chain</u>, a member of the team, devised the <u>freeze-drying</u> technique which was an important part of the purification process.

2) At first Florey and Chain <u>didn't</u> have the <u>resources</u> to produce penicillin in large amounts. They made penicillin for their first <u>clinical trial</u> by growing <u>Penicillium notatum</u> in every container they could find in their lab. Their patient began to recover, only to die when the penicillin <u>ran out</u>.

Florey took penicillin to America for Mass Production

Florey knew that <u>penicillin</u> could be vital in treating the <u>wounds</u> of soldiers fighting in World War II. British <u>chemical firms</u> were too busy making <u>explosives</u> to start mass production — so he went to <u>America</u>.

1) American firms were also not keen to help — until America <u>joined the war</u> in 1941. In December 1941, the US government began to give out <u>grants</u> to businesses that <u>manufactured</u> penicillin.

2) By 1943, British businesses had also started <u>mass-producing</u> penicillin. Mass production was sufficient for the needs of the <u>military medics</u> by 1944.

3) After the war, the <u>cost</u> of penicillin fell, making it more accessible for <u>general use</u>.

4) Fleming, Florey and Chain were awarded the <u>Nobel Prize</u> in 1945.

> Today, penicillin is used to treat a <u>range</u> of <u>bacterial</u> infections, including chest infections and skin infections. Other <u>antibiotics</u> were discovered after 1945, including treatments for lung infections, acne and bacterial meningitis.

Comment and Analysis

While <u>individuals</u> (like Florey, Chain and Fleming) were important in making the discovery of penicillin, it was large institutions like <u>governments</u> that funded its mass production.

Case Study: Penicillin

The discovery and mass production of penicillin were important developments in medicine — but they didn't happen overnight. Try these activities to make sure you know how the use of penicillin developed.

Knowledge and Understanding

1) What is penicillin and why is it important?

2) In your own words, explain how Fleming discovered penicillin. Use the key words below.

   culture dish   chance   fungal spore   mould   bacteria

3) Why was Fleming unable to advance his work once his findings were published?

4) Why was Florey and Chain's first clinical trial of penicillin unsuccessful? Give as much detail as you can.

Thinking Historically

1) Copy and complete the diagram below, explaining the consequence of each event on the development of penicillin. Try to include as much detail as possible.

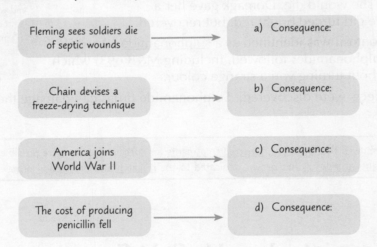

Fleming sees soldiers die of septic wounds → a) Consequence:

Chain devises a freeze-drying technique → b) Consequence:

America joins World War II → c) Consequence:

The cost of producing penicillin fell → d) Consequence:

2) What do you think was the significance of institutions in the success of penicillin? Use your answers from the question above as well as information from p.52.

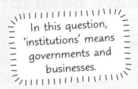

In this question, 'institutions' means governments and businesses.

3) Do you think the discovery of penicillin had more or less of an impact on medicine than Jenner's work on the smallpox vaccination? Use information from pages 32 and 52 to explain your answer.

EXAM TIP

Penicillin isn't just mould news — it's still used today...

You should write out a quick plan for the longer questions in the exam. This will help you not to miss out any key points and make your argument coherent and well structured.

Modern Treatments

Scientists have found a range of other treatments for diseases, besides penicillin.
These include magic bullets, which use chemical and synthetic substances to kill bacteria.

Paul Ehrlich discovered the first Magic Bullet — Salvarsan 606

Antibodies were identified as a natural defence mechanism of the body against germs. It was known that antibodies only attacked specific microbes — so they were nicknamed magic bullets. In 1889, Paul Ehrlich set out to find chemicals that could act as synthetic antibodies.

1) First, Ehrlich discovered dyes that could kill the malaria and sleeping sickness germs.

2) In 1905, the bacterium that causes the sexually transmitted disease syphilis was identified.

3) Ehrlich and his team decided to search for an arsenic compound that was a magic bullet for syphilis. They hoped it would target the bacteria without poisoning the rest of the body.

4) Over 600 compounds were tried, but none seemed to work.

5) In 1909, Sahachiro Hata joined the team. He rechecked the results and saw that compound number 606 actually appeared to work. It was first used on a human in 1911 under the trade name Salvarsan 606.

Gerhard Domagk found the second Magic Bullet — Prontosil

1) In 1932, Gerhard Domagk found that a red dye, prontosil, stopped the streptococcus microbe from multiplying in mice — without being poisonous to the mice.

2) In 1935, Domagk's daughter pricked herself with a needle and caught the disease. Afraid she would die, Domagk gave her a large dose of prontosil. The girl turned bright red, but recovered.

> Streptococcus caused blood poisoning which was often fatal, and which could be contracted from very minor wounds. Many surgeons contracted it after cutting themselves in the operating theatre.

3) The active ingredient of prontosil was identified as a sulphonamide. A whole group of drugs based on sulphonamides followed, including M&B 693, which worked on pneumonia without turning you a strange colour.

4) Sadly more serious side-effects were discovered. Sulphonamide drugs can damage the liver and kidneys.

Comment and Analysis

The discovery of magic bullets showed that synthetic, targeted treatments for specific diseases were possible. Since Paul Ehrlich's first discovery, a huge pharmaceutical industry has grown, dedicated to the research and production of new treatments.

Treatments have been introduced to fight Cancer

1) The first successful treatment against cancer that didn't involve surgery was radiotherapy, introduced after the discovery of radiation in 1896-1898 by Antoine Henri Becquerel, Marie Curie and Pierre Curie. Radiotherapy involves killing cancer cells using targeted X-rays and gamma rays.

2) Chemotherapy is the treatment of cancer using drugs. It was discovered in World War II when doctors found that nitrogen mustard (a chemical in mustard gas) could be used to reduce cancer tumours. Other drugs were later discovered, including a compound in folic acid that blocks the growth of cancer cells.

3) Since the late 1990s, targeted therapy has been used to fight cancer. This uses drugs to prevent cancer from spreading.

Modern Treatments

More names, more discoveries, more treatments — do these activities to make sure you've got them sussed.

Knowledge and Understanding

1) What is meant by the term 'magic bullet'?

2) Copy and complete the timeline below, summarising the events related to the discovery of Salvarsan 606. Try to give as much detail as you can.

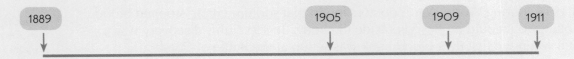

1889   1905   1909   1911

3) Copy and complete the table below about different cancer treatments.

Treatment	Description of treatment	When it was discovered
a) **Radiotherapy**		
b) **Chemotherapy**		
c) **Targeted therapy**		

Thinking Historically

1) Explain why you think the Germ Theory (p.34) was important for the discovery of Salvarsan 606 and Prontosil.

2) Copy and complete the mind maps below, listing the medical treatments used in the medieval period and medical treatments used in the 20th century.

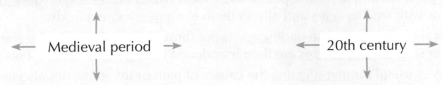

← Medieval period →   ← 20th century →

3) Using the mind maps above, compare how similar treatments were in these two periods.

EXAM TIP

When it comes to magic bullets, Ehrlich hit the mark...

In Paper 1, Section B, you'll only need to answer one of questions 5 or 6 — don't answer both questions. You should pick the question you feel you can give the strongest answer for.

c.1900-Present: Medicine in Modern Britain

Modern Surgery

Surgery improved rapidly during the 20th century. The discovery of <u>blood groups</u> made <u>blood transfusions</u> more successful, and even <u>heart transplants</u> are now possible. Nowadays the emphasis is on <u>precision</u>.

Blood Transfusions have solved the problem of Blood Loss

The idea of <u>blood transfusions</u> was known from the 17th century, but they were rarely successful because the blood of the recipient often <u>clotted</u>. Blood also clotted if it was stored <u>outside the body</u>.

1) In 1900, <u>Karl Landsteiner</u> discovered <u>blood groups</u>. <u>Certain blood groups</u> can't be mixed as the blood will clot, <u>clogging</u> the blood vessels. He found that transfusions were <u>safe</u> as long as the patient's blood <u>matched</u> the blood donor's.

2) In 1914, during World War I, doctors found that <u>sodium citrate</u> stopped blood clotting so it could be <u>stored</u> outside the body. In 1917, this discovery was vital when the first ever <u>blood bank</u> was set up at the Battle of Cambrai.

3) In 1946, the <u>British National Blood Transfusion Service</u> was established.

Patients always suffer some <u>blood loss</u> during <u>surgery</u>. If a lot of blood is lost, this can be <u>fatal</u>. Blood transfusions helped to <u>prevent</u> this cause of death by allowing surgeons to <u>replace</u> any blood lost during surgery.

Transplants have been made more Successful

1) In 1905, the first successful <u>transplant</u> of the <u>cornea of the eye</u> was performed. During the First World War, surgeons developed techniques for <u>skin transplantation</u>.

2) The first complete organ to be successfully transplanted was the <u>kidney</u>. <u>Livers</u>, <u>lungs</u>, <u>pancreases</u> and <u>bone marrow</u> can now also be transplanted.

3) The first successful <u>heart</u> transplant was carried out by the South African surgeon <u>Christiaan Barnard</u> in 1967. The patient only survived for <u>18 days</u> — he died of pneumonia.

The problem for transplants is <u>rejection</u>. The <u>immune system</u> attacks the implant as if it were a virus.
- The success of early transplant operations was limited because doctors lacked effective <u>immunosuppressants</u> — drugs that <u>stop</u> the immune system attacking.
- Since the 1970s, researchers have developed <u>increasingly effective</u> immunosuppressants, making transplants <u>safer</u> and more likely to be <u>successful</u>.

Keyhole Surgery and Robot-assisted Surgery increased Precision

1) <u>Keyhole surgery</u> is a technique (developed in the 1980s) which makes surgery <u>less invasive</u> — it leaves patients with smaller <u>scars</u> and allows them to <u>recover</u> more quickly.

2) A type of surgical camera called an <u>endoscope</u> is put through a <u>small cut</u>, letting the surgeon <u>see inside</u> the body. Other surgical <u>instruments</u> are then introduced through even smaller cuts in the skin.

3) Keyhole surgery is useful for <u>investigating</u> the causes of pain or infertility. It's also used for vasectomies, removing cysts or the appendix, mending hernias and other minor operations.

<u>Robot-assisted surgery</u> has also improved precision.
- The first <u>surgical robot</u> was introduced in 1985 but robot-assisted surgery only became widely used after 2000 with the launch of the da Vinci system.
- Robot-assisted surgery allows surgeons to make <u>smaller</u> cuts. This means less <u>scarring</u>, less <u>infection</u> and <u>quicker healing</u> of wounds.

These new types of surgery have made it <u>safer</u> for patients by limiting the possibility of <u>infection</u> and <u>blood loss</u>, as well as reducing the <u>shock</u> and <u>trauma</u> of surgery.

Modern Surgery

Surgery has become much safer thanks to developments in blood transfusions and keyhole surgery.
The following activities will help you understand the importance of these surgical developments.

Knowledge and Understanding

1) Explain why Karl Landsteiner's discovery of blood groups
   was important to the development of blood transfusions.

2) Explain the significance of the following in modern surgery:
   a) sodium citrate
   b) immunosuppressants

3) In your own words, explain what keyhole surgery is.

Thinking Historically

1) Which of the following do you think has had the biggest impact on
   modern medicine? Write a few sentences to explain your answer.

   > blood transfusions   transplants   keyhole and robot-assisted surgery

2) Copy and complete the table below, listing changes to surgery during
   c.1700-c.1900 (see pages 38 and 40) and changes from 1900 onwards.

Surgery in c.1700-c.1900	Surgery from 1900 onwards

3) Do you think there was a greater change in surgery during c.1700-c.1900 or
   from 1900 onwards? Explain your answer, using the table above to help you.

4) Copy and complete these mind maps, comparing the role of barber-surgeons (see page 12)
   and modern surgeons. You may want to include details about: knowledge and training, their
   contribution to medical developments and social attitudes to the profession of surgery.

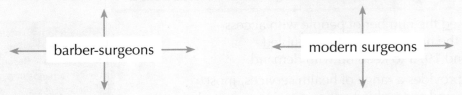

barber-surgeons   modern surgeons

All you need to do is transplant these facts into your brain...

*To hit the top marks on the last question of the paper, you need to go beyond the prompts
given in the question. You can use these as a starting point, but write about other factors too.*

c.1900-Present: Medicine in Modern Britain

The National Health Service

Advances in science and technology improved the <u>quality</u> of healthcare during the 20th century. But it was only with the founding of the <u>National Health Service</u> that <u>everyone</u> in Britain felt the benefits.

Before the NHS, access to Healthcare was Limited

1) At the start of the 20th century, access to healthcare was <u>severely limited</u>. This was particularly the case for <u>poor</u> people, who <u>couldn't afford</u> to go to the doctor or buy medicine.

2) This meant that people's health was poor. For example, in 1901 there were <u>140 infant deaths</u> for every 1000 births — today it's <u>less than 5</u>. When the <u>Boer War</u> broke out in 1899, army officers found that 40% of volunteers were <u>physically unfit</u> for military service.

3) In 1911, the Liberal government introduced the <u>National Insurance Act</u>, which gave some workers <u>health insurance</u> to pay for medical attention. But <u>World War I</u> drained Britain's resources, and several <u>economic slumps</u> in the 1920s and 1930s meant the government couldn't expand healthcare provision.

The NHS was established in 1948

1) The <u>Second World War</u> (1939-1945) changed people's <u>attitudes</u> towards healthcare:

- The raising of a mass army made powerful people <u>take notice</u> of the <u>health problems</u> of the poor.
- Air raids, especially the Blitz of 1940, prompted the government to set up the <u>Emergency Medical Service</u>. This provided a <u>centralised control</u> of medical services and offered <u>free treatment</u> to air raid casualties. It proved <u>successful</u> under great pressure.

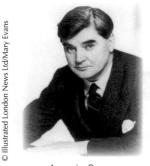

Aneurin Bevan.

2) In 1942, the social reformer <u>William Beveridge</u> published a <u>report</u>. The report called for government provision of social security <u>'from the cradle to the grave'</u>. The report became a <u>bestseller</u>.

3) In 1945, the <u>Labour Party</u> was elected with a mandate to implement Beveridge's proposals, primarily by founding the <u>National Health Service</u> (NHS) in <u>1948</u>.

4) <u>Aneurin Bevan</u> was the Minister for Health who introduced the NHS. Bevan wanted the NHS to be <u>free</u> at the point of use — he set up a system of compulsory <u>National Insurance</u> to pay for it.

5) Bevan wooed doctors and dentists with a <u>fixed payment</u> for each registered patient. They were also allowed to continue treating private fee-paying patients. By 1948 nearly <u>all hospitals</u> and 92% of <u>doctors</u> had joined the NHS.

Comment and Analysis

The founding of the NHS showed that <u>government intervention</u> could make a positive impact on people's health. However, it took a change in <u>public attitudes</u> (backed up by greater <u>scientific knowledge</u>) to make it happen.

The NHS has improved Access to Healthcare

1) The NHS <u>increased</u> the number of people with access to healthcare — the number of doctors <u>doubled</u> between 1948 and 1973 to keep up with demand.

2) Today, the NHS provides a range of health services, most of which are <u>free</u> and <u>accessible</u> to everyone. They include <u>accident and emergency</u> care, <u>maternity</u> care and major <u>surgery</u>, as well as <u>pharmacies</u>, <u>dentists</u>, <u>mental health</u> services, <u>sexual health</u> services and general practitioners (<u>GPs</u>).

> The NHS has encountered some <u>problems</u> in providing <u>access</u> to care. The 1980 Black Report suggested that the NHS <u>hadn't</u> improved the health of the very <u>poorest</u>. Patients also had to suffer <u>long waiting times</u> during the 1990s. In 2000 the government drew up an '<u>NHS plan</u>' to deal with waiting times among other areas.

The National Health Service

The NHS was a turning point in British healthcare — check you understand what you've read with this page.

Knowledge and Understanding

1) Copy and complete the table below, stating how each statistic is linked to healthcare and the year(s) it relates to.

Statistic	Link to healthcare	Year(s)
a) 140 out of 1000		
b) 40%		
c) 92%		
d) Doubled in number		

2) In your own words, describe how the following individuals affected British healthcare. Give as much detail as possible.

   a) William Beveridge

   b) Aneurin Bevan

Thinking Historically

1) Copy and complete the mind maps below, describing what health and healthcare was like for ordinary people in the Renaissance period and at the turn of the 20th century.

   ↑
   ← Renaissance period →
   ↓

   ↑
   ← Turn of the 20th century →
   ↓

2) Using your mind maps, explain the similarities between health and healthcare for ordinary people in these two periods.

3) Copy and complete the table below, listing the ways World War I and World War II affected medicine. You can include information from elsewhere in the section.

World War I	World War II

4) Do you think World War II was the main reason that the NHS was created? Use your answers to the questions above to help explain your answer.

Beveridge Report — it's not about your favourite drink...

When considering if one factor is more important than another, it's good to think about how many other things it impacts. The most important factors normally have many consequences.

The Government's Role in Healthcare

Since 1900, the <u>government's role</u> in improving people's health has <u>grown and grown</u>.

Vaccination Campaigns have eradicated some Diseases

Since 1900, the government has launched several national <u>vaccination</u> programmes to <u>prevent</u> people from catching deadly diseases. These have been <u>successful</u> in reducing the number of deaths from such diseases.

<u>Diphtheria</u> is a contagious disease that is caused by bacteria in the <u>nose</u> and <u>throat</u>. It can eventually attack the heart muscles, causing <u>paralysis</u> or <u>heart failure</u>.

- Before the 1940s, diphtheria was a major killer disease — in 1940, there were over <u>60,000 cases</u> of the disease and over <u>3,000 deaths</u>.

- After fears that wartime conditions could lead to the spread of the disease, the government started a <u>vaccination campaign</u> in 1940.

- The government ran <u>publicity campaigns</u>, using posters, newspaper advertisements and radio broadcasts.

- The campaign was a success — by 1957, the number of diphtheria cases had dropped to just <u>38</u>, with only <u>six deaths</u>.

> In 1940, the easiest way to reach children was through <u>schools</u>, so <u>5-15 year olds</u> were vaccinated ahead of the youngest children who were most vulnerable. The establishment of the <u>NHS</u> in <u>1948</u> (see p.58) allowed the government to vaccinate <u>all</u> children by their <u>first birthday</u>.

<u>Polio</u> is an infection that can attack the digestive system, bloodstream and nervous system. The disease can cause <u>paralysis</u>, and particularly affects <u>children</u>.

- In the late 1940s and early 1950s, Britain suffered a series of polio <u>epidemics</u> — the disease made over 30,000 children disabled between 1947 and 1958.

- The first vaccine was introduced in Britain in 1956 alongside a <u>national campaign</u>, aiming to vaccinate every person <u>under the age of 40</u>.

- The campaign was successful, with the disease all but <u>eradicated</u> by the late 1970s. In the period 1985-2002, only <u>40 polio cases</u> were reported in Britain.

Lifestyle Campaigns aim to improve people's Health

In the 20th century, scientists showed a link between people's <u>lifestyle choices</u> and their <u>health</u> (see p.48). The government ran several <u>campaigns</u> to make people aware of the dangers and to <u>change</u> their <u>lifestyles</u>.

1) In 1952, a <u>Great Smog</u> caused by coal fires resulted in <u>4,000 deaths</u> in London. It showed the dangers of <u>air pollution</u>, which can cause breathing conditions like <u>asthma</u> and <u>bronchitis</u>. The government passed laws in the hope of limiting air pollution.

2) An increase in <u>less active lifestyles</u> has led to an increase in <u>obesity</u>. In 2009, the government launched the <u>Change4Life</u> campaign, with the aim of <u>improving diets</u> and <u>promoting daily exercise</u>.

3) Excessive <u>alcohol</u> intake has been linked to several diseases, most notably <u>liver cirrhosis</u>. Alcohol intake <u>rose</u> between 1950 and 2004, but has since <u>fallen</u>. This may be due to the government's <u>Drinkaware</u> campaign, launched in 2004. The Drinkaware logo appears on many alcohol advertisements.

> **Comment and Analysis**
>
> These campaigns mark a <u>big shift</u> in the government's approach from the foundation of the NHS, and an even bigger shift from the <u>laissez-faire attitudes</u> of the 19th century, when people thought government shouldn't intervene at all in public health. Not only is the government trying to <u>treat</u> and <u>vaccinate against</u> known diseases, it is now <u>intervening in people's lives</u> in order to stop them getting particular illnesses in the first place.

The Government's Role in Healthcare

The government's role in healthcare is a lot different today to how it was in the past. These activities focus on the ways the government has had a significant impact on combatting disease in the last hundred years.

Knowledge and Understanding

1) Explain what the government did to try to prevent each of these diseases.

   a) Diphtheria   b) Polio   c) Liver cirrhosis

2) Which government campaign do you think was the most successful? Explain your answer.

3) How did the creation of the NHS improve the process of vaccination?

Thinking Historically

1) Why do you think Edward Jenner was important for the eradication of diphtheria and polio? Use information from page 32 to explain your answer.

2) Copy and complete the mind map below, writing as much detail as you can about government involvement in healthcare during these time periods.
   You can use the information on page 62 and previous pages to help.

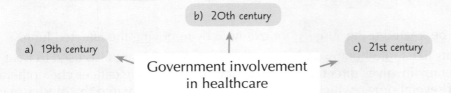

b) 20th century

a) 19th century   Government involvement in healthcare   c) 21st century

3) In which century do you think the government had the most significant effect on healthcare? Explain your answer.

4) 'The creation of the NHS was the most important development in British medicine in the period c.1900-present.' Use the table to help you structure each paragraph of an essay explaining how far you agree with this view.

Point	Evidence	Why evidence supports point?
Landsteiner's discovery of blood groups was an important development in British medicine during c.1900-present.	The discovery of blood groups led to blood transfusions, which made surgery safer. It also meant blood tests could be run to diagnose a range of diseases with more accuracy.	The developments made due to the discovery of blood groups have meant that patients are treated earlier, more effectively and more safely. This has saved many lives and greatly increased our understanding of disease.

Add three rows to the table to plan three more paragraphs.

Make sure your write points that agree and disagree with the statement.

Talk about different factors from this time period.

My free speech campaign is getting everybody talking...

There are many examples of the government's role in healthcare — e.g. their vaccination campaign against diphtheria. Don't just give examples though, explain why they're important.

c.1900-Present: Medicine in Modern Britain

Case Study: Lung Cancer

Lung cancer is a disease that was much more common after 1900 than before. The battle against lung cancer is an example of science and technology and government campaigns working side by side.

Lung Cancer can be caused by Smoking

1) Lung cancer was a rare disease in 1900, but became common by the 1940s. Today, around 20% of all cancer deaths in the UK are due to lung cancer. Approximately 43,500 people are diagnosed every year.

2) Scientists have estimated that around 90% of lung cancer cases can be linked to tobacco smoking. The popularity of smoking increased in the First World War, particularly among soldiers. Smoking soon became popular among women too.

3) In 1950 the link between smoking and lung cancer was proven by Richard Doll and Austin Bradford Hill.

Lung cancer Diagnostics and Treatment have Improved

Advances in science and technology have made it easier to diagnose and treat lung cancer.

- Chest X-rays are the first means of diagnosing lung cancer. The X-rays can't show whether the patient definitely has cancer, but can show if there is anything on the lung that shouldn't be there.
- CT scans (see p.50) can be used to give a more detailed image of the lungs.
- Doctors can now use bronchoscopy to diagnose lung cancer. This involves putting a thin tube into the lungs to take a sample of the suspected cells. It requires a local anaesthetic to numb the throat.

- Lung cancer can be treated using surgery, for example by removing the affected lung.
- Modern treatments like radiotherapy and chemotherapy (see p.54) are also used to treat lung cancer. Radiotherapy involves directing radiation at the lungs. Lung cancer chemotherapy uses a combination of several drugs, which are normally injected directly into the bloodstream.

Government Campaigns have reduced smoking

When the link between smoking and lung cancer became clear, the government warned people of the risks.

1) In 1962 the Royal College of Physicians recommended a ban on tobacco advertising. Shortly afterwards, in 1965, cigarette adverts were banned from television. In 1971 tobacco companies were forced to put a health warning on cigarette packets.

2) In recent years, the government has put a ban on smoking in public places — this was introduced in Scotland in 2006, and in England and Wales in 2007.

3) Recent government campaigns have focused on helping people to give up smoking and on discouraging smoking in cars, homes and in front of children.

4) In March 2015 Parliament passed a law requiring all cigarette companies to use plain packaging on boxes of cigarettes.

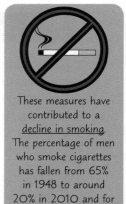

These measures have contributed to a decline in smoking. The percentage of men who smoke cigarettes has fallen from 65% in 1948 to around 20% in 2010 and for women it's dropped from 41% to 20% in the same period.

Comment and Analysis

Lung cancer prevention is a good example of an area of health where the government has been increasingly active — the large number of television campaigns and pieces of legislation show that the government is now taking health seriously, which is in contrast to its attitude before 1900.

Case Study: Lung Cancer

This page will help your understanding of the actions taken to reduce the impact of lung cancer.

Knowledge and Understanding

1) Who proved the link between smoking and lung cancer?

2) In your own words, give three ways science and technology
   have made it easier to diagnose and treat lung cancer.

3) Copy and complete the timeline below by filling in all of the key events
   which contributed to a decline in smoking. Give as much detail as possible.

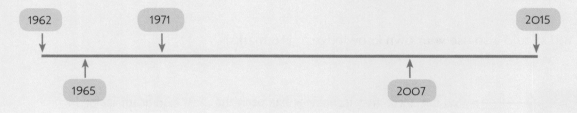

| 1962 | 1971 | 2015 |

| 1965 | 2007 |

Thinking Historically

1) Copy and complete the table below, describing the similarities and differences in
   the responses to Doll and Bradford Hill's discovery, and John Snow's discovery
   (see page 42) about the link between cholera and contaminated water.

Similarities	Differences

2) Think about the discoveries from the question above. Which discovery do you
   think prompted the biggest government response? Give reasons for your answer.

3) Copy and complete the mind maps below, explaining the ways that institutions and individuals
   have tried to cure and prevent disease since c.1900. Use ideas from the whole of this section.

← Cure disease →   ← Prevent disease →

4) Do you think there has been more emphasis on curing disease
   or preventing disease since c.1900? Explain your answer.

Dreams of a healthy lifestyle went up in smoke...

*Think about what people would have known at the time. The link between lung cancer and
smoking seems obvious now, but it wouldn't have been known to people in the early 1900s.*

c.1900-Present: Medicine in Modern Britain

Worked Exam-Style Question

The sample answer below will help you with the 16-mark question in the exam.

'Technology has been the most significant factor in the development of medicine in Britain since c.1500.'

Explain how far you agree with this statement.

You could mention:
- Antonie van Leeuwenhoek
- X-rays

You should also use your own knowledge.   [16 marks]

> It's a good idea to include a short introduction summarising your argument.

I do not agree that technology has been the most significant factor in the development of health and medicine in Britain since c.1500. Although technology has had a major impact on medicine since the 1800s, other factors were more important in earlier periods.

> This paragraph explains why technology has been significant.

Technology was important to the development of medicine in the 1800s as it allowed people to make new medical discoveries. Louis Pasteur's discovery that germs cause disease (published as the Germ Theory in 1861) was made possible by developments in microscope technology. The microscope was invented by Antonie van Leeuwenhoek in the 17th century and improved designs were created in the 1800s. These improvements allowed Pasteur to see clear images of germs for the first time.

> Use specific and relevant examples to support your points.

> Explain how the factor in the question had an impact on medicine's development

> Include specific dates to show you have a good knowledge of the period.

Technology has also been significant in improving diagnosis and treatment, especially in the late 1800s and the 1900s. The invention of diagnostic technology like X-rays (discovered in 1895) and CT scans (invented in 1972) has allowed doctors to diagnose illnesses more effectively and intervene before a disease becomes too advanced. For example, X-rays and CT scans have both been used to improve the diagnosis of lung cancer. Since the 1980s, new technology, like the endoscope, has led to the development of keyhole surgery. This allows surgeons to be more precise and use smaller cuts when operating, which means that patients recover more quickly and with less risk of infection. Technological advances like these have had a huge impact on the development of health and medicine by improving the ability of surgeons and doctors to diagnose patients and provide safer and more effective treatment.

> You need to show you know the order of events.

Worked Exam-Style Question

Even if you agree with the statement, it's important to consider both sides of the argument.

However, before the 1800s, other factors were more important to the development of medicine. For example, in the Renaissance period, the advancement of medical knowledge was a key factor in the development of medicine. Many doctors began to use dissection and experimentation in this period to improve their understanding of the human body. Vesalius' work on human anatomy laid the foundations for improvements in diagnosis and treatment of disease, while Sydenham's observation of symptoms allowed him to develop more effective treatments for many ailments, including the use of iron to treat anaemia.

Don't just focus on the factor in the question — you should also write about other factors.

You should include examples from throughout your answer.

Start a new paragraph every time you introduce a new factor.

Technology did have a minor impact on the development of medicine in the Renaissance period. For example, William Harvey's discovery that blood circulated around the body was informed by new technology — his ideas about the function of the heart were inspired by the way a new type of water pump worked. The invention of the printing press also allowed new ideas like those of Vesalius to be shared. However, technology was not the most important factor in this period.

Explain how each point you make is relevant to the question.

Moreover, while technology has been important since the 1800s, it cannot be considered the most important factor because it has often required economic investment from large institutions like the government in order to have an impact. For example, since the mid-20th century, access to modern medical technology like MRI scans and ultrasounds has relied on funding from the National Health Service. Founded in 1948, the NHS provides free access to a range of medical services, including expensive medical equipment. This demonstrates that technology has mainly had an impact on the development of medicine when it is supported by the economic resources of large institutions like the government.

Remember to explain the significance of each factor you write about.

Make sure you give a clear answer to the question in your conclusion.

In conclusion, technology has not been the most important factor in the development of medicine in Britain, because before the 1800s other factors, such as advances in medical knowledge, were more important. Even though technology has had a major impact on health and medicine since the 1800s, it is still not the most significant factor, because its impact in this period has relied on other factors, especially government funding.

Summarise your argument in your conclusion.

c.1900-Present: Medicine in Modern Britain

Exam-Style Questions

Give these exam-style questions a go to test your knowledge of modern medicine.
Remember that you might need to include details about medicine from earlier periods too.

Exam-Style Questions

1) Explain one similarity between government involvement in
   healthcare in the 20th century and the period c.1700-c.1900.   [4 marks]

2) Explain why there were changes in surgery between the
   end of 19th century and the end of the 20th century.

   You could mention:
   - the discovery of blood groups
   - World War I

   You should also use your own knowledge.   [12 marks]

3) 'Alexander Fleming's discovery of penicillin was the
   most important moment in medicine since c.1800.'

   Explain how far you agree with this statement.

   You could mention:
   - the development of magic bullets
   - the discovery of DNA

   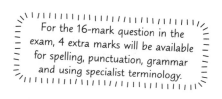
   For the 16-mark question in the
   exam, 4 extra marks will be available
   for spelling, punctuation, grammar
   and using specialist terminology.

   You should also use your own knowledge.   [16 marks]

Exam-Style Questions

Exam-Style Questions

4) Explain one difference between hospitals in the 20th century and hospitals in the medieval period (c.1250-c.1500).   [4 marks]

5) Explain why ideas about the causes of disease changed significantly in Britain between the end of the 19th century and today.

You could mention:
- the discovery of DNA
- lifestyle factors

You should also use your own knowledge.   [12 marks]

6) 'The government was the most important factor in the improvement of people's health in Britain since c.1250.'

Explain how far you agree with this statement.

You could mention:
- the NHS
- the development of vaccinations

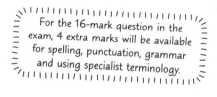
For the 16-mark question in the exam, 4 extra marks will be available for spelling, punctuation, grammar and using specialist terminology.

You should also use your own knowledge.   [16 marks]

The British Sector of the Western Front, 1914-1918

Trench Warfare on the Western Front

So that's the thematic study done and dusted. Now it's on to the historic environment section. Between 1914 and 1918, the Allies (including Britain, France and Belgium) fought the German Imperial Army in Belgium and France — the area where the fighting happened was called the Western Front.

The War on the Western Front was mostly Fought in Trenches

In the autumn of 1914, the Germans and the Allies realised that they couldn't beat each other outright. Instead of retreating, they built a line of trenches that stretched through northern France to the coast of Belgium. These trench lines were developed throughout the war, but their position mostly stayed the same.

1) In July 1916, the British tried to break through the German line in an area called the Somme — lots of lives were lost during this offensive.

2) In 1917, mines were used at Arras and Ypres to break through the enemy line (see p.70) — the aim was to avoid losses like those at the Somme by making it easier for the infantry to attack the enemy trenches.

3) The army also tried to improve medical care after the casualties of the Somme overwhelmed medical staff. In 1917, more medical posts were set up to prepare for casualties before a big offensive on the Ypres Salient.

During the Third Battle of Ypres, from July to November 1917, there were over 200,000 casualties. This time, there were 379 Medical Officers, so many men were treated earlier than those at the Somme.

A salient is where one side's line pushes into the other side's line — their territory gets surrounded by the enemy on three sides.

4) By April 1917, the Germans had retreated to the Hindenburg line. In November 1917 at the Battle of Cambrai, the Allies broke its defences with tanks, but they lost this ground again later. There were about 45,000 British casualties — fewer than at the Somme, but still a high number.

Before the Battle of Cambrai, a blood bank was set up by Captain Robertson (see p.78) — he realised that it would be easier to save lives during the battle if they had a ready supply of blood.

On the first day of the Battle of the Somme, there were almost 60,000 British casualties — 20,000 of these were killed. There were only 174 Medical Officers treating tens of thousands of serious casualties in the first week of the battle. Many men died because they had to wait for days before being treated.

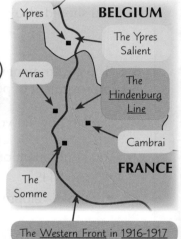

Ypres
BELGIUM
The Ypres Salient
Arras
The Hindenburg Line
Cambrai
FRANCE
The Somme

The Western Front in 1916-1917

Trenches were Designed to Protect Soldiers from Enemy Attack

1) Most trenches were dug down into the ground and their upper level was fortified with sandbags. In wet areas, trenches were built upwards using sandbags full of clay — these were called 'breastworks'. Ideally, trenches were about six or seven feet deep.

2) Trenches were constructed by 'entrenching' (lots of soldiers in a line digging straight into the ground), 'sapping' (one man digging outwards from the end of the trench) or 'tunnelling' (like sapping, but a layer of earth was left along the top of the trench until it was finished).

Mounds of earth were built from the side of the trench to split it into sections — these were called 'traverses'.

The floors of trenches in wet areas were often lined using wooden boards called 'duckboards'.

The parapet was built up in a similar way to the parados on the front side of the trench. It was meant to be bulletproof, and was lined with wooden planks, netting or sandbags.

Barbed wire was set in front of the trench to make it harder for enemy infantry to attack head on.

The parados was a mound of earth or sandbags that raised the height of the back of the trench. It was designed to protect soldiers from shell explosions behind the trench.

The ground between the front line trenches of each side was called 'no man's land'.

Fire trenches (trenches closest to the enemy) had a firing step, held back by wooden planks — men could stand on here behind the bulletproof parapet and fire their rifles into no man's land.

To the enemy trenches.

Trench Warfare on the Western Front

Have a go at the activities below about medical provision at the Somme and the construction of trenches.

Source Analysis

The sources below were both produced during the Battle of the Somme.
Source A comes from the diary of a British nurse. Source B is a photograph of soldiers who were wounded in the battle waiting to be transported to a hospital.

Source A

Thursday, July 6 1916: In ordinary times we get a telegraph from Abbeville saying a train with so many on board has left and is coming to us. Then they stopped giving numbers — just said "full train". Now not even a telegram comes — but the full trains do. Yesterday, in addition to our 1300 beds we took over the lounge of a large restaurant, the orderlies' barracks, the ambulance garage, the Casino front and part of the officers' mess.

Source B

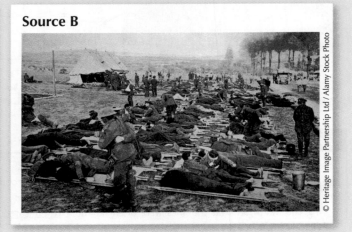

© Heritage Image Partnership Ltd / Alamy Stock Photo

1) Copy and complete the table below by explaining how the content, authorship and date of Source A affect its usefulness for an investigation into the provision of medical care during the Battle of the Somme.

Feature	Usefulness
a) **Content**	
b) **Author**	
c) **Date written**	

2) Imagine you are using Source B for an investigation into the provision of medical care during the Battle of the Somme. Explain how each feature on the right influences the usefulness of the source for your investigation.

a) Content

b) Type

Knowledge and Understanding

1) Using your own words, explain three things the British Army did to reduce casualties and improve medical care after the Battle of the Somme in 1916.

2) Explain three different techniques that were used to construct trenches.

3) Without looking at page 68, draw a diagram of a trench. Label its main features and explain the purpose of each one.

EXAM TIP

Trench warfare was new to everyone...

Avoid making general statements about the usefulness of sources. Instead, think about the specific features of each source that make it useful for the investigation you've been given.

Trench Warfare on the Western Front

Trench systems were expanded during the war — this had a big impact on the terrain of the Western Front.

Trenches were often Organised in Parallel Lines

Fire trench

Supervision trench

According to one 1916 training manual, trenches were ideally built in three parallel lines.

'Saps' were small trenches that pushed out into no man's land.

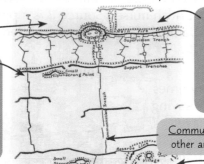

The front line had two trenches. The 'fire trench' faced the enemy. The 'supervision trench' was used to move along the line behind the fire trench. They had zig-zag or step-shaped sections separated by traverses (p.68). This stopped enemy infantry from firing along the trench, and contained explosions from shells in small areas.

The 'support trench' was about 60 to 90 metres behind the front trench — this protected it from shell bombardment aimed at the front line. It was connected to the front line trench by communication trenches — soldiers could retreat to the support trench, and the support trench reinforced the front line.

Communication trenches connected the trench lines to each other and to local roads and army depots behind the lines.

Comment and Analysis

This image shows an ideal trench system. In reality, building such organised trenches was hard — they might be built quickly as troops advanced. Terrain had to be considered too. Trench maps drawn during the war show that the lines were often far more complicated.

The 'reserve trench' was about 350 to 550 metres behind the front line. It was made up of dugouts (shelters that protected 4 to 6 men) or lines of trenches. Reinforcements waited here so they could counter enemy attacks.

Underground Warfare was a Key Feature of the Western Front

Both sides tunnelled under no man's land to reach enemy trenches. It was dangerous for tunnellers, who could be buried, suffocate or meet the enemy, but it was less costly than a normal infantry attack through no man's land.

In 1916, the Allies built a tunnel network under Arras by extending existing caves, quarries and mines — it had electricity, accommodation and a hospital (p.72). In April 1917, it was used to hide 24,000 men before the Battle of Arras. Tunnels were dug up to the German line so men could reach the enemy trenches in safety — the entrances were blown open with mines at the start of the battle. Lots of ground was won on the first day. However, the British suffered over 150,000 casualties during the battle.

At the Battle of Messines on the Ypres Salient in June 1917, 19 mines were blown up under the German line. Around 10,000 German soldiers died instantly. Two of the mines were used to destroy defences on hills — Hill 60 and the Caterpillar. They would have been hard to attack head on without heavy losses.

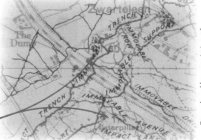

Reproduced by permission of the National Library of Scotland.

A trench map of Hill 60 and the Caterpillar in April 1917. German trenches are red and British are blue.

Comment and Analysis

Trench maps are a good source for studying the layout of trenches and their defences. They're more realistic than the ideal layout in training manuals. They were drawn up using photos taken from the air. Teams on the ground collected information too. They don't always give the full picture, though. For example, machine gun placements were often deliberately hidden and could be missed by planes.

Trench Warfare damaged Terrain and Transport Networks

1) Shelling and entrenchment damaged roads and terrain on the Western Front. The British army used motor and horse-drawn vehicles to move supplies towards the Front from 'supply dumps' near railway lines, but the muddy, shell-damaged terrain was hard to negotiate. Railways became important for moving supplies and troops around behind the front lines, but they weren't always near the Front.

2) It was hard to evacuate wounded men from the front lines quickly. Stretcher bearers often had to carry casualties down communication trenches or through a series of relay posts — this delayed wound treatment.

By 1917, the British had built a light railway network behind the lines (other Allied armies had done this already). This made it easier to move supplies, ammunition and men through muddy and damaged terrain, and to evacuate wounded men from the Front.

Trench Warfare on the Western Front

There's a lot of content on the previous page, so have a go at these activities to make sure you've understood everything and can use it to help you answer the source-based questions in the exam.

Knowledge and Understanding

1) Without looking at page 70, draw a diagram of a trench system. Label the different kinds of trench, explain the purpose of each one and describe their key features.

2) Using your own words, describe how the Allies used underground warfare at the Battle of Arras and the Battle of Messines.

3) Why was it difficult to evacuate wounded men from the front lines quickly?

4) Why did it become easier for the British Army to evacuate wounded men by 1917?

Source Analysis

The source below is a photograph taken during the Battle of Arras in April 1917. Some details in the source have been highlighted.

a) Many injured soldiers are waiting to be moved.

b) The terrain is muddy and shell-damaged.

c) Stretcher bearers are struggling on the difficult terrain.

© Imperial War Museum (Q 3216)

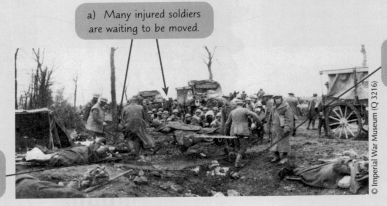

1) Copy and complete the table below. For each detail, write down a question that you could ask to find out more about the impact trench warfare had on transport networks on the Western Front. Then, give an example of the type of source that might help you to answer each question and explain how the source would be useful.

Detail	Question	Useful source	How the source would be useful
a) Many injured soldiers are waiting to be moved.			
b) The terrain is muddy and shell-damaged.			
c) Stretcher bearers are struggling on the difficult terrain.			

I'll never complain about potholes again...

The first question in the exam is all about describing features. To get full marks, you'll need to identify two separate features and give a piece of supporting information about each one.

The British Sector of the Western Front, 1914-1918

The RAMC and the FANY

The fighting on the Western Front <u>disrupted local transport networks</u>. The British Army were supported by various <u>medical units</u> who treated wounded men and <u>evacuated</u> them from the front line.

The Royal Army Medical Corps (RAMC) ran Field Ambulances

1) <u>Moving casualties</u> away from the Front to be treated was a problem — the terrain had become very <u>muddy</u>.

2) The RAMC Field Ambulances (these were <u>units</u>, not vehicles) set up <u>mobile medical stations</u>. <u>Stretcher bearers</u> carried casualties through a series of <u>relay posts</u> until they reached a medical post or somewhere they could be moved by <u>road</u>, <u>rail</u> or <u>river</u>.

Field Ambulance <u>transport</u> included:
- Teams of <u>stretcher bearers</u>.
- <u>Horses</u>, <u>wagons</u> and <u>carts</u>.
- <u>Motor ambulances</u> (the RAMC started using these in <u>1915</u>).

The RAMC Field Ambulances created the Chain of Evacuation

Men were <u>more likely to survive</u> if their wounds were <u>treated quickly</u>. The RAMC developed a <u>system</u> to move wounded men who had a <u>chance of surviving</u> to medical areas — this was called 'the <u>Chain of Evacuation</u>'.

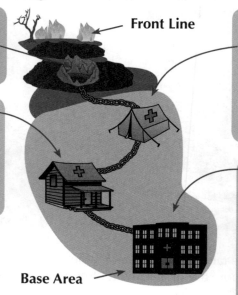

Front Line

Base Area

A <u>Regimental Aid Post (RAP)</u> was set up a few metres behind the <u>front line</u> in a shell hole or dugout. They gave <u>first aid</u>. Men who needed more treatment <u>walked</u> or were <u>carried</u> by stretcher bearers to an <u>Advanced Dressing Station</u>.

<u>Casualty Clearing Stations</u> collected seriously injured men from Main Dressing Stations using <u>motor ambulance convoys</u>. They had <u>surgical</u> and <u>medical</u> wards in <u>wooden huts</u>, <u>nursing staff</u>, and were sometimes supported by <u>mobile X-ray units</u> (see p.78 for more on X-rays). Men could be treated for up to <u>four weeks</u> before being moved to a <u>Base Hospital</u> or sent back to the Front.

The army prepared for the <u>Battle of Arras</u> in 1917 by setting up a <u>hospital</u> with room to treat <u>700 men</u> in the <u>Arras tunnels</u> (p.70). It had an <u>operating theatre</u>, waiting rooms for the wounded, and rest areas for stretcher bearers.

<u>Advanced Dressing Stations</u> were ideally set up around 350 metres from the RAP in <u>tents</u>, <u>dugouts</u> or <u>large buildings</u>. <u>Main Dressing Stations</u> were set up about <u>1 mile</u> behind the Advanced Dressing Stations. They collected injured men from the RAP using <u>horse-drawn ambulances</u> and <u>stretcher bearers</u>. Seriously injured men were moved to <u>Casualty Clearing Stations</u>.

<u>Base Hospitals</u> were designed to take up to <u>400</u> patients. They were often turned into <u>specialist hospitals</u> to treat common injuries and ailments (e.g. the effects of <u>gas</u>). They were set up in <u>large buildings</u> and were often close to <u>transport networks</u>. They also had <u>X-ray departments</u>. They treated patients until they could be sent back to the Front or <u>sent home</u> to Britain.

The FANY provided Transport Services to the Allied Armies

1) The <u>women</u> of the <u>First Aid Nursing Yeomanry Corps</u> (FANY) were trained in <u>first aid</u>, <u>veterinary skills</u>, <u>signalling</u> and <u>driving</u>. They mainly worked as a <u>field ambulance</u>, moving wounded men between base hospitals, medical posts, trains, barges and hospital ships. The FANY staffed two key <u>ambulance convoys</u> — the Calais Convoy and the St. Omer Convoy.

One FANY driver called <u>Beryl Hutchinson</u> who was part of the <u>St. Omer Convoy</u> described her role in her <u>memoirs</u>. She had to <u>pick up wounded men</u> from <u>trains</u> and drive them to <u>base hospitals</u> or to <u>boats</u> that would take them back to <u>Britain</u>. The <u>driving skills</u> of the FANY were pretty useful when it came to transporting men who were <u>very badly wounded</u> — they had to drive as <u>smoothly</u> as possible so that the men wouldn't be jolted around. <u>Canal barges</u> were used to move the <u>worst cases</u>.

The <u>driving skills</u> of the FANY were very <u>useful</u> to the army, as they needed to <u>move</u> supplies, wounded men and rations between <u>coastal ports</u> and the <u>front line</u>.

2) The FANY had many roles. They ran a mobile <u>soup kitchen</u> and a mobile <u>bathing vehicle</u>, staffed <u>hospitals</u> and <u>convalescent homes</u>, ran a hospital <u>canteen</u> and organised <u>concerts</u> for the troops.

The RAMC and the FANY

Try these activities to practise using details from a source to come up with your own historical questions, and to improve your knowledge of the Chain of Evacuation.

Source Analysis

The source below is from the autobiography of R.C. Sherriff, an officer in the British Army who was injured at the Third Battle of Ypres in 1917.

1) Some details in the source have been underlined. For each detail, write down a question you could ask to find out more about dressing stations in the British Army's Chain of Evacuation. The first one has been done for you.

a) Why did injured soldiers have to 'drag' themselves to dressing stations?

c)

The company commander took one look at us and said, "Get back as best you can, and find a dressing station"... Here and there were other walking wounded... <u>Many were so badly wounded that they could barely drag themselves along</u>, but to save themselves was their only hope. There was no one else to save them... It seemed <u>hours before we reached a dressing station</u>, then <u>only by a lucky chance</u>. It was a <u>ramshackle tin shelter</u> amid a dump of sandbags that once had been a gun emplacement... <u>The doctor swabbed the wounds on our hands and faces</u> and tried to see through the holes in our uniforms where pieces had gone in. "You don't seem to have got anything very deep," he said. "Can you go on?"

b)

d)

2) For each of the questions, give an example of a source that could be used to answer it. Explain how the source would help you to answer the question.

Look at page 80 for some examples of types of sources.

Knowledge and Understanding

1) The diagram below shows the Chain of Evacuation. Copy and complete it by adding the name of each stage in the chain and a description of its role.

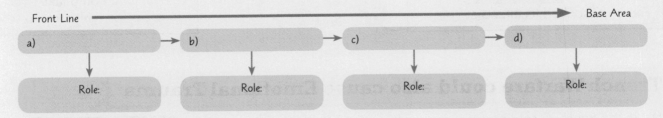

Front Line ⟶ Base Area

a)   b)   c)   d)

Role: Role: Role: Role:

2) In your own words, explain the role of the following groups on the Western Front:
   a) Royal Army Medical Corps (RAMC)
   b) First Aid Nursing Yeomanry Corps (FANY)

The army really liked their acronyms...

When you write a historical question in the exam, you'll start by picking out a detail from the source to follow up on. Make sure your question is clearly linked to the detail you've chosen.

Conditions in the Trenches

Life in the trenches exposed soldiers to lots of <u>illnesses</u> and <u>infections</u> — they were also at risk of <u>gas attacks</u>.

Bad Conditions in the Trenches caused Illness

1) Soldiers were exposed to the <u>weather</u> in the trenches. Many suffered from <u>exposure</u> to the cold and <u>frostbite</u>, especially in the cold winter of <u>1916-17</u>.

2) <u>Trench foot</u> was a condition caused by standing in <u>flooded trenches</u> for too long. Skin and tissue on the feet <u>broke down</u>. It could become <u>gangrenous</u> (infected) — doctors used <u>amputation</u> to stop the <u>gangrene</u> from spreading.

3) <u>Dysentery</u> caused <u>diarrhoea</u> and <u>dehydration</u>. <u>Dirty water</u> and unhygienic <u>latrines</u> (holes about 4 or 5 feet deep that served as <u>toilets</u>) helped this disease to spread.

4) The trenches were also full of <u>vermin</u> that <u>spread diseases</u>, like rats, lice, maggots and flies. <u>Trench fever</u> and <u>typhus</u> were spread by body lice — it could take <u>12 weeks</u> to <u>recover</u>.

> Trench foot was more common at the <u>start</u> of the war. By <u>1915</u>, there were fewer cases, as soldiers had to change their <u>socks</u> frequently. They also put <u>whale oil</u> on their feet to create a <u>waterproof</u> layer.

> Doctors didn't make the link between <u>lice</u> and <u>trench fever</u> until <u>1918</u>. <u>Delousing stations</u> were set up to try and <u>stop</u> outbreaks of these diseases, but they weren't always <u>successful</u>. It was hard to remove <u>lice eggs</u> from soldiers' clothing.

Both sides used Gas Attacks to Disable Soldiers

<u>Four main types</u> of gas were <u>weaponised</u> during the war — the <u>effects</u> of each could be <u>devastating</u>.

Lachrimatory Gas — from 1914

Also known as <u>tear gas</u>. It caused <u>inflammation</u> of the nose, throat and lungs, and <u>blindness</u>. It was meant to <u>disable</u> soldiers or force them to <u>retreat</u>, rather than <u>kill them</u>.

Mustard Gas — from July 1917

A '<u>blistering agent</u>' that caused blisters, burning and breathing difficulties. Extended exposure to mustard gas could cause <u>blindness</u> and <u>lung infections</u>. It ate away at the body from the <u>inside</u>, and it could take up to <u>five weeks</u> to die. The gas could cling to <u>clothes</u> for hours, which put <u>medical staff</u> at risk too.

Chlorine Gas — from April 1915

Chlorine gas was the first <u>deadly gas</u> used on the Western Front. It was a '<u>killing agent</u>' that <u>slowly suffocated</u> its victims. A <u>medical officer</u> for the French described its effects at <u>Ypres</u>.

> "...I felt the action of the gas on my <u>respiratory system</u>; it <u>burned</u> in my throat, caused <u>pains</u> in my chest, and made <u>breathing</u> all but impossible. I <u>spat blood</u> and suffered from <u>dizziness</u>. We all thought we were lost."
> (April 1915)

Phosgene — from December 1915

This gas caused <u>suffocation</u>. Phosgene had a mild <u>scent</u> and was <u>colourless</u>, so it was hard to detect. It could take over <u>24 hours</u> for symptoms to set in.

Trench Warfare could also cause Emotional Trauma

1) In the trenches, soldiers were exposed to lots of <u>death</u>, <u>destruction</u> and <u>artillery bombardment</u>. Living in these harsh conditions could cause a <u>psychological illness</u> called <u>shell shock</u>.

2) <u>Symptoms</u> of <u>shell shock</u> could include tiredness, blindness, hearing loss, shaking and <u>mental breakdown</u>. Doctors disagreed over whether it was caused by <u>unseen physical injuries</u> or by <u>emotional trauma</u>.

Comment and Analysis

'<u>Shell shock</u>' meant <u>two different things</u>:

1) When an <u>explosion</u> shocked the central nervous system, causing <u>brain damage</u>.

2) An <u>emotional disorder</u> caused by the <u>traumatic</u> trench environment.

> After the <u>Battle of the Somme</u> in <u>1916</u>, there was an <u>increase</u> in shell shock cases — doctors started to evacuate these cases to <u>specialist hospitals</u>. However, the <u>emotional trauma</u> caused by <u>trench warfare</u> wasn't really understood until later in the war — even then, many with shell shock were seen as <u>cowards</u>.

Conditions in the Trenches

This page will help you revise the most common health problems on the Western Front and their causes.

Knowledge and Understanding

1) Copy and complete the table below by explaining the causes of different health problems experienced by soldiers on the Western Front.

Health problem	Cause(s)
a) Frostbite	
b) Trench foot	
c) Diarrhoea and dehydration	
d) Trench fever and typhus	
e) Shell shock	

2) Make a set of flashcards to help you learn the different types of gas that were used as weapons during the war. On one side, write the name of the gas and when it was first used. On the other side, without looking at page 74, write the effect that the gas had and any other information that you can remember about it.

Source Analysis

The source below is from the medical case records of a British soldier who was sent to The National Hospital, Queen Square in London because he was suffering from shell shock. It was written in 1915.

> Patient had a great deal to do with handling wounded and dying soldiers which made a deep impression on him... The noises made by shells and the uncertainty of where they would strike caused great uneasiness and strain. Patient's comrades remarked that he did not answer when they spoke to him and appeared not to realize that they were speaking to him. Of this he knew nothing until told later on. He could not hold his weapon properly, nor shoot accurately. He was very shaky. Suffered much from headache. He was sent away from trenches November 14 and arrived at Southampton November 21.

1) In the boxes below, there are three investigations about shell shock on the Western Front. Which investigation do you think the source above would be most useful for? Explain your choice.

a) How effective were treatments for shell shock during WWI?	b) How well was shell shock understood by the end of WWI?	c) What were the symptoms of shell shock?

2) Why do you think the source would be less useful for the other two investigations?

The trenches were pretty horrific...

It's really important that you know how trench warfare affected soldiers' health, so make sure you learn about all the different health problems covered on page 74 and what caused them.

The British Sector of the Western Front, 1914-1918

Wounds and Injuries

Trench warfare caused <u>horrific injuries</u> on a <u>scale</u> doctors had not seen before the war.

Soldiers were often Wounded by Gunfire and Shell Explosions

1) Machine guns and rifles caused <u>gunshot wounds</u>, bruises, fractured bones and organ damage.

2) Trenches often protected the <u>body</u>, but the <u>head</u> was <u>exposed</u> — the army were alarmed at the <u>number</u> and <u>severity</u> of <u>head injuries</u>. They saw injuries like shrapnel embedded in the brain, <u>skull fractures</u>, large scalp cuts and <u>brain damage</u>. In 1915, metal 'Brodie' helmets were issued. Before this, many head injuries were <u>fatal</u>. The helmets gave soldiers a <u>better chance</u> of surviving, but treatment was still limited.

   > American surgeon <u>Dr Harvey Cushing</u> treated <u>head injuries</u> during the war. He pioneered <u>new surgical techniques</u> that were still being used in the <u>1970s</u>. His techniques <u>halved</u> the number of deaths caused by brain surgery during the war. He used <u>X-rays</u> to find <u>shrapnel in the brain</u> and drew it out using <u>magnets</u>. His efforts were limited by <u>slow evacuation</u> and lack of <u>brain imaging techniques</u>.

3) <u>Shrapnel</u> (metal objects and fragments from explosions) caused horrific <u>facial injuries</u> and could <u>kill instantly</u>. <u>Shrapnel shells</u> were blown open <u>in the air</u> using a small fuse — they were filled with <u>bullets</u> and <u>metal balls</u> which <u>flew out</u> and hit soldiers. Other shells were designed to <u>explode violently</u> — the cases of these <u>high explosive shells</u> broke into large <u>jagged</u> pieces of shrapnel that <u>tore</u> through flesh.

   > Dr Harold Gillies, a <u>British surgeon</u>, treated <u>serious facial injuries</u> at Queen Mary's Hospital in Sidcup during and after the war. He developed a <u>plastic surgery</u> technique called the <u>tube pedicle</u>, which made <u>skin grafting</u> and <u>facial reconstruction</u> more effective.

4) Soldiers could also get <u>concussions</u> from <u>shell explosions</u>, be hit by flying debris, buried under collapsed buildings and trenches or <u>poisoned</u> by carbon monoxide from blasts which then collected in air pockets.

Wound Infection was a Big Problem

1) Many trenches were dug in <u>farmland</u>, which was covered in bacteria from <u>fertilisers</u>. In Flanders, <u>drainage ditches</u> had been destroyed by <u>shelling</u>, so trenches were often <u>waterlogged</u> and <u>bacteria thrived</u>.

2) The ground was also infected by <u>unhygienic latrines</u> and <u>thousands of bodies</u> that were left to <u>decompose</u> or were buried in <u>shallow graves</u> near the trenches.

3) Wounded men often had to lie in the <u>contaminated mud</u> of trenches or no man's land for <u>hours</u> or <u>days</u> before being picked up by stretcher bearers. They were at risk of getting <u>serious infections</u> like <u>tetanus</u> and <u>gas gangrene</u> — these were <u>fatal</u> without treatment. Infections could also cause <u>sepsis</u>.

> "...there were numerous dug outs, and these so <u>filthy</u> that our men could not occupy them, the bottom of the <u>trenches were paved with dead</u> all German so far as we could learn, and very <u>badly decomposed</u>..."
> Extract from the 10th Canadian Battalion's war diary describing conditions in a French trench on the Ypres Salient in April 1915.

> "...<u>every gunshot wound</u> of this war in France and Belgium is more or less <u>infected</u> at the moment of its infliction... <u>mud and dirt</u> pervade everything; and bacteriological investigations of the <u>soil</u>, of the <u>clothing</u>, and of the <u>skin</u> demonstrate the presence of the most <u>dangerous pathogenic organisms</u> in all three."
> Extract from a 1916 lecture by British Army surgeon Sir Anthony Bowlby.

Comment and Analysis

Doctors like Bowlby realised that <u>every wound</u> was likely to be <u>infected</u>. This was a <u>big problem</u> for the army, as those with only <u>minor injuries</u> were still at risk of dying from a <u>fatal infection</u>.

There were a Few Ways to Fight Infection at the Start of the War

1) <u>Anti-tetanus serum</u> was given to <u>injured soldiers</u> on the front line to <u>prevent</u> tetanus.

2) Wounds were <u>thoroughly washed</u> in an <u>antiseptic</u> solution called <u>carbolic lotion</u>, <u>closed up</u> and wrapped in <u>bandages soaked</u> in carbolic acid.

3) A <u>paraffin paste</u> called <u>Bipp</u> was used to <u>cover wounds</u> to <u>prevent</u> infection.

4) Before <u>antibiotics</u> were discovered in the 1920s, <u>amputation</u> of <u>wounded</u> arms, legs, hands or feet was a common way to stop <u>life-threatening infections</u> from spreading.

Wounds and Injuries

The activities below are all about the wounds and injuries that soldiers suffered on the Western Front.

Knowledge and Understanding

1) Copy and complete the mind map below about head and facial injuries on the Western Front.

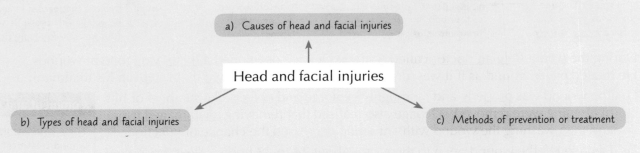

a) Causes of head and facial injuries

Head and facial injuries

b) Types of head and facial injuries

c) Methods of prevention or treatment

2) In your own words, give three reasons why soldiers' wounds were likely to become infected on the Western Front.

3) Explain how each of the following methods was used to fight wound infection:
   a) Anti-tetanus serum
   b) Carbolic lotion
   c) Bipp
   d) Amputation

Source Analysis

The source below is an extract from the medical case records of a soldier who suffered a gunshot wound to the head while serving on the Western Front. He was evacuated to a hospital in Newcastle, where the source was written by medical staff on 26 July 1915.

> The patient says he received the wound on 9th July 1915 at Camill about 10.30 am. He "lost his senses" for 15 minutes. He walked down to the dressing station (2 miles) and he lay till 1 am till moved by the motor ambulance and he was taken to... the clearing station... He was operated upon. Operation: "An area of almost the size of 2/6 piece* was removed... Cleaned and drained. Wound was very septic before the operation."

*A large coin

1) Imagine you are using this source for an investigation into the treatment of head injuries on the Western Front. Explain how each feature of the source listed below affects its usefulness for your investigation.

   a) Author   b) Date   c) Purpose   d) Content

I'm feeling a bit squeamish now...

For question 2(a) in the exam, you'll have two different sources to write about. Remember that you should write about each one separately — you don't need to compare them.

The British Sector of the Western Front, 1914-1918

Developments in Surgery and Medicine

During the war, doctors developed <u>new techniques</u> for dealing with <u>serious injuries</u> and <u>infections</u>.

The number of Deaths from Wound Infection was Reduced

In the <u>19th century</u>, surgeons tried to avoid <u>germs</u> getting into wounds — this was called <u>aseptic surgery</u>.	They started to <u>disinfect</u> their hands <u>before</u> surgery and wear <u>surgical gloves</u>. They also <u>sterilised</u> their operating theatres and instruments to get rid of germs.	<u>Antiseptics</u> like carbolic acid were used to kill germs and prevent wound infection.	However, <u>wound treatment</u> was still very basic before the war. Doctors quickly <u>explored</u> the wound for objects that needed removing, then <u>washed the wound</u> with antiseptic and sewed it up (this was called <u>primary closure</u>).

During the war, a <u>Belgian doctor</u> called <u>Antoine Depage</u> developed a <u>better way</u> to treat wounds. He treated every wound as if it was <u>already infected</u>. There were <u>two main steps</u> in his treatment:

1) The wound was <u>properly</u> and <u>thoroughly explored</u> and <u>objects</u> like shrapnel or bits of clothing were removed. Depage also realised that removing <u>all damaged tissue</u> and <u>then</u> washing the wound with antiseptic <u>decreased</u> the chance of <u>infection</u>.

2) Depage left the wound <u>open to the air</u> for about 24 to 48 hours. Next, he looked at a <u>swab</u> of the wound under a microscope to check for bacteria. If the wound <u>wasn't infected</u>, then he closed it up — this was called <u>delayed primary closure</u>.

> In <u>1915</u>, <u>Alexis Carrel</u> and <u>Henry Dakin</u> developed a new way to <u>prevent infection</u>. <u>Dakin</u> created an <u>antiseptic solution</u> that could be flushed into a wound using rubber tubes <u>before</u> closure — this technique was called <u>irrigation</u>. <u>Depage</u> used this method as part of his wound treatment.

Comment and Analysis

These <u>improvements</u> in wound treatment <u>saved</u> many men from having <u>amputations</u> just to stop infections from <u>spreading</u>. Allied surgeons also used these techniques to improve the <u>chances of surviving</u> an amputation.

Fracture Treatment was improved by X-Rays and Splints

1) Wilhelm Roentgen discovered <u>X-rays</u> in <u>1895</u>. During the war, hospitals used <u>X-ray machines</u> to find <u>broken bones</u> and <u>shrapnel</u>.

2) The British had <u>528 X-ray units</u> — <u>14</u> of these were <u>mobile units</u>. They took <u>mobile X-ray machines</u> and <u>radiographers</u> to <u>casualty clearing stations</u>, so men could be treated <u>closer</u> to the front line.

Before <u>X-ray machines</u>, surgeons had to look for shrapnel by hand, putting their patients at risk of <u>infection</u>. X-ray machines made aseptic surgery <u>more effective</u>, because the surgeon didn't have to <u>touch</u> the wound to find shrapnel and bone fragments.

3) At the start of the war, <u>80%</u> of men who suffered a <u>fractured femur</u> (thigh bone) in the trenches <u>died</u>. A <u>surgeon</u> called Robert Jones treated this injury using the <u>Thomas splint</u>.

4) The <u>Thomas splint</u> was strapped around the broken leg <u>before</u> the casualty was moved. This stopped the leg from moving, so that it was <u>protected</u> from more damage. By <u>1915</u>, only <u>20%</u> of soldiers with this kind of injury <u>died</u>.

In <u>1917</u>, Robert Jones released a book (influenced by his war experience) <u>advising doctors</u> in Britain on how to treat complicated shoulder, leg, arm, spinal and pelvic <u>fractures</u>. It explained how to use <u>splints</u> to treat certain fractures.

Blood Transfusions were used to treat Blood Loss

1) <u>Blood loss</u> caused many deaths during the war. British doctors <u>transfused</u> blood from one person to another (<u>direct transfusion</u>), but it was a <u>slow process</u> and not always successful.

2) A <u>new method</u> called the <u>syringe-cannula technique</u> was developed. Doctors took blood from a <u>donor</u> using a <u>needle</u> and <u>syringe</u> and transfused it into their patient <u>quickly</u>. It was tricky to carry out, as blood could <u>clot</u> in the syringe.

3) In <u>1917</u>, a US Army doctor called <u>Captain Oswald Robertson</u> argued that it would be better to collect blood <u>before it was needed</u>. As a result, the first <u>blood bank</u> was set up in preparation for the <u>Battle of Cambrai</u> in <u>1917</u>.

In <u>1914</u>, it was discovered that adding <u>sodium citrate</u> to blood stopped <u>clotting</u> so it could be <u>stored</u>. In <u>1916</u>, blood was added to a <u>citrate glucose solution</u>, so it could be stored on ice for about 10 to 14 days.

Developments in Surgery and Medicine

The activities below will help you learn about how the Western Front influenced surgery and medicine.

Knowledge and Understanding

1) Copy and complete the table below about the doctors and scientists who contributed to medical developments during the First World War.

Name	Technique they developed	What it was used for	How it worked
a) **Antoine Depage**			
b) **Alexis Carrel and Henry Dakin**			
c) **Robert Jones**			

2) In your own words, explain why X-ray machines were important for treating injuries caused by trench warfare.

3) The diagram below lists three problems related to blood transfusion. Explain how each problem was solved during the First World War.

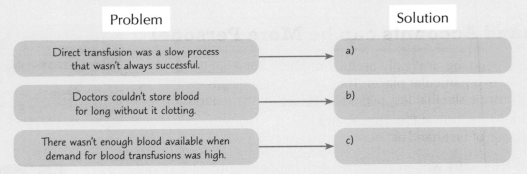

Problem — Solution

Direct transfusion was a slow process that wasn't always successful. → a)

Doctors couldn't store blood for long without it clotting. → b)

There wasn't enough blood available when demand for blood transfusions was high. → c)

Source Analysis

The source on the right is from an article in a medical journal, written by Captain Oswald Robertson. It was published in June 1918.

Imagine you are using this source for an investigation into the problem of blood loss on the Western Front.

1) How does the date of the source affect its usefulness for your investigation?

2) How does the author of the source affect its usefulness for your investigation?

> The effect of transfusion with preserved blood was fully as striking as that observed after the giving of freshly drawn blood. There was the same marked improvement in colour, the pulse became slower and stronger, and the blood pressure showed an increase of 20 to 40 points.

 EXAM TIP

War doctors set the stage for modern medicine...

It's important to learn the names of key figures, as well as information on why they're significant. It'll help you to support your answers with specific details in the exam.

The British Sector of the Western Front, 1914-1918

Types of Sources

When you're talking about the <u>usefulness</u> of sources, it's a good idea to think about what that source <u>can</u> and <u>can't tell you</u>. Some types of sources will give you <u>information</u> that other types of sources <u>don't</u>.

Different Types of Document have different Uses

Documents are <u>written sources</u> that contain <u>information</u> or <u>evidence</u>.

1) <u>Documents</u> like <u>official records</u> or <u>government reports</u> are useful if you're looking for <u>statistics</u> or <u>factual information</u> about your <u>site</u> and the <u>people</u> who used it.

2) There's often a <u>date</u> attached to <u>official documents</u> too, so you can tell exactly <u>when</u> the source was written. This is useful if you're looking for <u>evidence</u> that's linked to a <u>particular time</u> in your site's history.

3) Documents can be quite <u>one-sided</u>, and it's not always obvious <u>who wrote them</u>, so it can be hard to decide how <u>reliable</u> they are. This affects how <u>useful</u> the source is, as it's <u>hard to judge</u> how reliable the <u>facts</u> in the document are.

<u>Documentary sources</u> for the Western Front include diaries, letters, medical records, official reports written by RAMC and army officers, hospital admission records and government reports.

Documents
- Official Records
- Government Reports
- Diaries and Letters

4) <u>Record collections</u> are useful if you're trying to <u>spot patterns</u> or work out <u>how typical</u> a piece of evidence you've found might be. Lots of records are based on <u>forms</u> that ask for <u>certain facts</u> or <u>information</u> about a person, so they're really useful for <u>comparing the experiences</u> of different people.

Field Ambulance <u>hospital admission records</u> were based on forms. They sometimes used a <u>wound classification code</u> to show what type of wound a soldier had — these records are useful for working out which kinds of wounds were the <u>most common</u>.

First-hand Accounts can be More Personal

A <u>trench map</u> can't tell you what it <u>felt</u> like to be on the <u>front line</u>, but a <u>diary entry</u> or <u>memoir extract</u> that <u>describes</u> life at the Front can give a <u>really good idea</u> of <u>how it felt</u>. Personal accounts can be <u>one-sided</u>, though, so they're only useful as evidence of the experiences of <u>the person who wrote them</u>.

1) <u>First-hand accounts</u> are really useful for finding out <u>what it was like</u> to live in a particular place. They often <u>reveal details</u> about a historic site that <u>less personal sources</u> don't mention.

2) It's important to look at the <u>date</u>, <u>author</u> and <u>purpose</u> of first-hand accounts.

- A diary entry written <u>as events were happening</u> might be more <u>accurate</u> than a memoir or autobiography <u>written years later</u>, as it's easy to forget details, or focus on some more than others.

- An <u>official account</u> has a <u>different purpose</u> to a <u>personal account</u>. They're more useful if you're looking for <u>technical details</u> or if you want to know about the <u>priorities</u> of the <u>people in charge</u>.

First-hand Accounts
- Diaries or Memoirs
- First-hand Reports
- Autobiographies
- Oral Accounts

Image Sources can Show what a site Looked Like

1) <u>Maps</u> and <u>plans</u> are useful sources for looking at <u>how</u> a site was <u>laid out</u> and <u>organised</u>. Maps covering <u>large areas</u> are useful for putting the site into a <u>wider context</u>. Maps of a specific part or physical feature of a site can give a <u>detailed picture</u> of how the site <u>looked</u> and <u>worked</u>.

2) <u>Photos</u> give a <u>snapshot</u> of what a historic site looked like at a particular time. Photos don't always tell the <u>whole story</u>, though. Every photograph is taken by a <u>photographer</u> who <u>chooses</u> what to <u>focus on</u> and what to <u>leave out</u>.

Some photos of soldiers on the Western Front were <u>posed</u> so that <u>journalists</u> could use them in <u>magazines</u>. They showed an <u>idealised version</u> of life in the trenches. When you're <u>analysing</u> a photo to decide how <u>useful</u> it is, it's a good idea to use your <u>own knowledge</u> to decide whether it's giving a <u>typical</u> or <u>accurate</u> picture.

Image Sources
- Photographs
- Maps
- Plans
- Diagrams
- Artwork

Types of Sources

Try these activities to help you revise the different types of sources and how they can be used.

Knowledge and Understanding

1) Copy and complete the table below by listing some examples of each
type of source and then explaining their strengths and weaknesses.

Type of source	Examples	Strengths	Weaknesses
a) **Documents**			
b) **First-hand accounts**			
c) **Image sources**			

Source Analysis

Source A below comes from the official War Diary of the 44th Field Ambulance — a British medical unit operating on the Western Front. It describes the medical training activities of some new recruits.

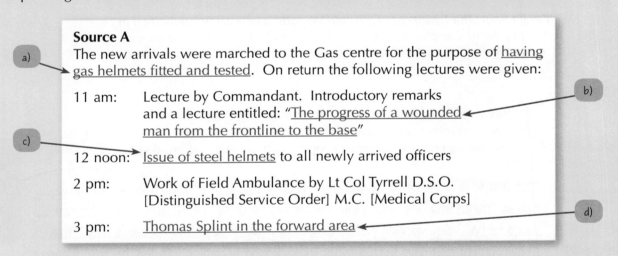

Source A

a) The new arrivals were marched to the Gas centre for the purpose of having gas helmets fitted and tested. On return the following lectures were given:

11 am: Lecture by Commandant. Introductory remarks and a lecture entitled: "The progress of a wounded man from the frontline to the base" b)

12 noon: Issue of steel helmets to all newly arrived officers c)

2 pm: Work of Field Ambulance by Lt Col Tyrrell D.S.O. [Distinguished Service Order] M.C. [Medical Corps]

3 pm: Thomas Splint in the forward area d)

1) Some details in the source have been underlined. For each detail, write down a question you could ask to find out more about the work of Field Ambulance units on the Western Front.

2) For each of your questions, give an example of a source that could be used to answer it. Explain how the source would help you to answer the question.

Some sources are more useful for putting on chips...

Your historical question should help you to find out more about the investigation you've been given, it shouldn't just be about random fact checking (e.g. "Was the author a fan of ketchup?")

The British Sector of the Western Front, 1914-1918

Worked Exam-Style Questions

The worked answers below will help you write your own answers to the source questions in the exam.

Source A

April 23: Soaking wet working in sap. Germans blew another mine this morning.
April 24: In wet sap again working past the knees in water and
water coming down your back like a shower bath. After about three
hours air so bad that we had to come out — candles would not burn.
April 27: Germans sent over gas shells which burst 200 yards away. Sent out thick
yellow smoke which rolled along like a fog bank, the wind driving it away. Went to
doctor to see about a cut on the ankle. He said it was septic and sent me to hospital.
April 28: In hospital. Plenty of company, wounded coming in all the time.

*From the war diary of John French, written in 1916. French survived
his time in hospital and had returned to the trenches by May 22.*

Source B

That the septic character of wounds is disastrous is also well known. During
the early hours, or the first few days, the wound is exposed to the danger of
gas-producing infection*. Later are developed the various infections, which,
either in the seat of fracture, in joints laid open, or in extensive lacerations** of
soft parts, sometimes give rise to lesions*** leading to amputation or to death.

*gas gangrene   **deep cuts   ***wounds

*Extract from 'The Treatment of Infected Wounds', a manual first published in
1916 by Alexis Carrel and Georges Dehelly to help doctors treating patients
on the Western Front. Carrel worked as a surgeon during the First World War.*

How useful are Sources A and B for studying the problem
of wound infection on the Western Front? Use both sources
and your own knowledge to support your answer. [8 marks]

> Always make
> it clear which
> source you're
> talking about.

> Use the
> question
> wording
> to show
> that you're
> answering
> it directly.

Source A is useful for studying the problem of wound infection because it gives
us an insight into how wound infections could occur on the Western Front. French
says he had been 'working past the knees in water' in saps into no man's land. This
environment may have been a factor in his wound becoming infected, because many
trenches were dug in farmland contaminated with bacteria from fertilisers. This
contamination was made worse by unhygienic latrines and dead bodies that were
often left to decompose or buried in shallow graves near the trenches.

> Use
> evidence from
> the source to
> support the
> points that
> you've made.

Source A is also useful because each diary entry is dated, and this shows that
French received treatment for his infected wound quickly — he saw a doctor on
27th April and was in hospital the next day. However, the usefulness of Source A
is limited because, as a diary entry, it only shows one man's experience of wound
infection and his case may not have been typical. It only took one day for French's

> Think about
> whether the
> information
> in the source
> is typical of
> other people's
> experiences.

> Consider
> the effect
> that the
> source type
> has on its
> usefulness.

Worked Exam-Style Questions

wound to be treated, but it could take much longer for casualties to receive medical care, especially during major battles. For instance, during the first week of the Battle of the Somme, there were only 174 Medical Officers treating tens of thousands of injured soldiers. This meant that many casualties had to wait for days to be treated, which could allow serious infections to develop. Source A is useful as it gives us some information about the causes and treatment of wound infection on the Western Front. However, the usefulness of the source is limited as it only represents the case of one soldier, whose experience was probably very different from that of soldiers who were injured in battle.

Source B is useful for studying the problem of wound infection because it explains that its consequences could include serious illnesses like gas gangrene, as well as amputation or even death. This reflects wider worries on the Western Front — it was 'well known' among doctors that every wound could get infected in the mud and dirt of the trenches. The source is useful because it not only tells us about the risks of wound infection, but also tells us that worries about the consequences were widespread among doctors.

The source was written by Alexis Carrel, who worked with Henry Dakin in 1915 to develop a new way of treating infected wounds called irrigation. Carrel was therefore an expert on the problem of wound infection on the Western Front, which makes the information he gives more reliable. Carrel wrote the source as a first hand account in 1916 when the war was still ongoing, informing doctors about the problems of infection that he had actually witnessed on the front. This makes the source more likely to be accurate, and therefore more useful for studying the problems of wound infection.

How could you further investigate Source A to learn more about the problem of wound infection on the Western Front?   [4 marks]

Detail from Source A to investigate: 'Went to doctor to see about a cut on the ankle. He said it was septic and sent me to hospital.'

Question you would ask: Was infection in small wounds a big issue for hospitals on the Western Front?

Type of source you might use: Hospital admission records for a hospital near the Western Front, saying why each soldier was admitted to hospital.

How this could help answer the question: This source would show how common it was for soldiers to be admitted to hospital with small infected wounds, which would help me to see how much pressure this put on Western Front hospitals.

The British Sector of the Western Front, 1914-1918

Exam-Style Questions

Here are some exam-style questions for the Historic Environment part of your exam for you to get stuck into.

Source A

An extract from a lecture given by W.H. Rivers to the Royal School of Medicine in 1917. Rivers was a psychiatrist who worked with shell-shocked soldiers, like the patient he is discussing here.

> On admission into hospital he suffered from fearful headaches and had hardly any sleep, and when he slept he had terrifying dreams of warfare. When he came under my care two months later his chief complaint was that, whereas ordinarily he felt cheerful and keen on life, there would come upon him at times, with absolute suddenness, the most terrible depression... which he could only describe as "something quite on its own".

Source B

'Gassed', a painting produced by John Singer Sargent in 1918-1919. It shows soldiers who have been blinded in a gas attack. Sargent was a 'war artist', which meant he was sponsored by the British government to visit the Western Front and record images of the First World War.

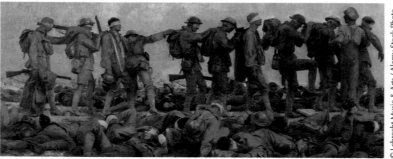

© Lebrecht Music & Arts / Alamy Stock Photo

Exam-Style Questions

1) Give a description of two features of Base Hospitals on the Western Front. [4 marks]

2) How useful are Sources A and B for studying the impact of trench warfare on soldiers on the Western Front? Use both sources and your own knowledge to support your answer. [8 marks]

3) How could you further investigate Source A to learn more about the impact of trench warfare on soldiers on the Western Front? Write down:
   a) A detail from Source A to investigate.
   b) A question you would ask.
   c) A type of source you might use.
   d) How this could help answer the question. [4 marks]

Answers

Marking the Activities

We've included sample answers for all the activities. When you're marking your work, remember that our answers are just a guide — a lot of the activities ask you to give your own opinion, so there isn't always a 'correct answer'.

Marking the Exam-Style Questions

For each exam-style question, we've covered some key points that your answer could include. Our answers are just examples though — answers very different to ours could also get top marks.

Most exam questions in history are level marked. This means the examiner puts your answer into one of several levels. Then they award marks based on how well your answer matches the description for that level.

To reach a higher level, you'll need to give a 'more sophisticated' answer. Exactly what 'sophisticated' means will depend on the type of question, but, generally speaking, a more sophisticated answer could include more detail, more background knowledge or make a more complex judgement.

Start by choosing which level your answer falls into. If different parts of your answer match different level descriptions, then pick the level description that best matches your answer as a whole. A good way to do this is to start at 'Level 1' and go up to the next level each time your answer meets all the conditions of a level. Next, choose a mark. If your answer completely matches the level description, or parts of it match the level above, give yourself a high mark within the range of the level. If your answer mostly matches the level description, but some parts of it only just match, give yourself a mark in the middle of the range. Award yourself a lower mark within the range if your answer only just meets the conditions for that level or if parts of your answer only match the level below.

On this page, you can find the level descriptions for questions in the Thematic Study section of the exam. The level description for the Historic Environment section can be found on page 109.

Level descriptions:

4-mark questions:

Level 1 1-2 marks	The answer gives a simple description of one similarity/difference between features in the two periods. Some knowledge and understanding of the periods is shown.
Level 2 3-4 marks	The answer explains one similarity/difference between features in the two periods. Detailed knowledge and understanding is used to support the explanation.

12-mark questions:

Level 1 1-3 marks	Limited knowledge and understanding of the periods is shown. The answer gives a simple explanation of change/continuity. Ideas are generally unconnected and don't follow a logical order.
Level 2 4-6 marks	Some relevant knowledge and understanding of the periods is shown. The answer contains a basic analysis of reasons for change/continuity. An attempt has been made to organise ideas in a logical way.
Level 3 7-9 marks	A good level of knowledge and understanding of the periods is shown. The answer explores multiple reasons for change/continuity. It identifies some relevant connections between different points, and ideas are generally organised logically.
Level 4 10-12 marks	**Answers can't be awarded Level 4 if they only discuss the information suggested in the question.** Knowledge and understanding of the period is precise and detailed. The answer considers a range of reasons for change/continuity and analyses each one. All ideas are organised logically and connections between different points are identified to create a developed analysis of the topic.

16-mark questions:

Level 1 1-4 marks	The answer shows limited knowledge and understanding of the period. It gives a simple explanation of one or more factors relating to the topic. Ideas aren't organised with an overall argument in mind. There is no clear conclusion.
Level 2 5-8 marks	The answer shows some knowledge and understanding of the period. There is some analysis of how different factors relate to the topic. Ideas are organised with an overall argument in mind, but the conclusion isn't well supported by the answer.
Level 3 9-12 marks	The answer shows a good level of knowledge and understanding of the period, which is relevant to the question. It analyses how several different factors relate to the topic. Most ideas are organised to develop a clear argument and a well-supported conclusion.
Level 4 13-16 marks	**Answers can't be awarded Level 4 if they only discuss the information suggested in the question.** The answer shows an excellent level of relevant knowledge and understanding of the period. It analyses in detail how a range of factors relate to the topic. All ideas are well organised to develop a clear argument and a well-supported conclusion.

Answers

c.1250-c.1500: Medicine in Medieval England

Page 7 — Disease and the Supernatural

Knowledge and Understanding

1 a) People prayed and repented for their sins.
  b) Suspected witches were tried and executed.
  c) Exorcisms were performed by members of the Church to remove the evil spirits.

2 Doctors owned an almanac that gave them information about the position of planets and stars. They used this to help them diagnose the causes of a patient's illness by looking at how different star signs affected certain parts of their body.

Thinking Historically

1 a) The Church taught people that disease was a punishment from God for sinful behaviour. This encouraged people to pray and repent to try to cure their diseases.
  b) The Church promoted Galen's ideas about the human body. His work fit the Christian belief that God made human bodies and designed them to be perfect, so the Church made it central to medical teaching.
  c) The Church outlawed dissection, which meant doctors weren't allowed to investigate the human body themselves. Instead, they had to learn Galen's incorrect ideas that were based on animal dissection.

2 You can choose any option, as long as you explain your answer. For example:
  • The belief that disease was a punishment from God prevented medical development because it discouraged people from finding new cures. People thought their only options were to pray and repent.

3 You can choose either option, as long as you explain your answer. For example:
  • Astrology was significant in changing medieval attitudes to the causes of disease. Although we know that astrology cannot be used to diagnose a patient, it did suggest that medieval people were looking beyond religious reasons for the causes of disease.

Page 9 — Rational Explanations

Knowledge and Understanding

1 a) The Four Humours Theory was created by Hippocrates in Ancient Greek times. It said that the body was made up of four humours — blood, phlegm, yellow bile and black bile. In order to maintain good health, the humours need to be in balance.
  b) Galen thought diseases could be treated using opposites. He believed that an excessive amount of the humour that was causing a disease could be balanced out by giving the patient a food, drink, herb or spice related to the opposite humour.

2 A cold was thought to be caused by too much cold, wet phlegm, so a doctor might have told a patient with a cold to drink wine because it was considered to have hot and dry properties. Doctors thought this would balance out the humours that had caused the cold.

3 a) The miasma theory originated in Ancient Greece and Rome.
  b) The miasma theory says that bad air, which comes from anything that creates a bad smell such as an abattoir, causes disease.

  c) It was replaced by the Germ Theory in the 1860s.

4 The miasma theory encouraged people to clean the streets and do other hygienic things to prevent bad air. This sometimes helped stop the spread of disease.

Thinking Historically

1 a) Because the teachings of Galen and Hippocrates had been accepted for so long, people were unwilling to question their work. This meant that people didn't try to make their own discoveries about medicine.
  b) The Roman Catholic Church was extremely influential and powerful during the medieval period, so any medical texts approved by the Church were considered the absolute truth. This meant that it was very difficult to question any of their teachings.
  c) Medieval doctors followed Galen's ideas about anatomy because they weren't allowed to perform their own dissections. As Galen only ever dissected animals, his ideas on human anatomy were incorrect. This meant that medieval doctors had wrong ideas about the human body.

2 You can choose either option, as long as you explain your answer. For example:
  • Hippocrates and Galen were the most important influences on medieval medicine. Their teachings provided two of the most popular theories about the causes of disease at the time, the Theory of the Four Humours and the miasma theory. Furthermore, their ideas were studied centuries after their deaths, which meant their teachings were practised throughout the medieval period.

Page 11 — Treating Disease

Knowledge and Understanding

1 • Repentance — Flagellants whipped themselves in public to show God they were sorry, as they thought disease was a punishment from God.
  • Pilgrimage — People believed they could be cured by travelling to holy shrines.
  • Bloodletting — If a patient was diagnosed as having 'excess blood', a small cut or leeches were used to remove blood from the body. This treatment was developed due to the Four Humours Theory.
  • Purging — To remove excess humours from the body, a patient was given laxatives to make them excrete fluids.
  • Purifying the air — Physicians carried posies or oranges to protect themselves from inhaling 'bad air'.
  • Remedies — Early natural medicines that were made from herbs, spices, animal parts and minerals could be bought from an apothecary, a local wise woman or made at home.
  • Lucky charms — Some people used remedies based on superstitions, such as carrying lucky charms containing 'magical' ingredients like 'powdered unicorn horn'.
  • Superstitious treatments — Doctors might say certain words when providing treatment in order to make it more effective.

2 Medieval doctors continued to use bloodletting because they believed so strongly in the Four Humours Theory, they thought that removing blood from the body would help balance their humours. Their belief in the work of Galen and Hippocrates meant they overlooked the evidence that bloodletting was at best ineffective and at worst, fatal.

Answers

Thinking Historically

1 Belief in the Four Humours Theory led to treatments that removed fluids from the body, such as bloodletting and purging. These techniques were ineffective and often harmed the patient. Belief in the miasma theory meant people 'purified' the air. Physicians did this by carrying posies or oranges, and some people burnt juniper, myrrh and incense so smoke and scents would prevent disease from spreading. This treatment was ineffective because people were more focused on treating the air rather than the patient.

2 a) Evidence for — The belief that disease was a punishment from God meant prayer and repentance were common treatments.
   Evidence against — Some treatments were based on non-religious theories, such as bloodletting, which was based on the rational Four Humours Theory.

   b) Evidence for — Remedies were made from herbs, spices, animal parts and minerals.
   Evidence against — Medical treatments based on religion, such as prayer, came from spiritual beliefs rather than things found in the natural world.

   c) Evidence for — Some treatments were dangerous. For example, bloodletting caused more deaths than it prevented.
   Evidence against — Some treatments caused no harm to the patient, for example carrying a lucky charm.

3 You can choose either option for each statement, as long as you explain your answer. For example:

   a) • Religion was very influential in the medieval period — prayer and repentance were two major treatments. Medieval people also sometimes went on pilgrimages or whipped themselves. They used these treatments in order to please God in the hope that he would cure them. Religious treatments dominated medicine in the medieval period.

   b) • Medieval people frequently used things they found around them to make medical treatments. Remedies were made from herbs, spices and animal parts. Other important treatments of the time also used things found in nature — for example, posies and oranges were used to stop 'bad air', and leeches were used for bloodletting.

   c) • Most medieval medical treatments tended to cause more harm than good. For example, flagellants caused harm by whipping themselves and people were more likely to die from bloodletting than to be cured by it.

Page 13 — Treating Disease

Knowledge and Understanding

1 Physician:
   • Physicians were male doctors who trained at university for at least seven years, but had little practical experience.
   • They read ancient texts and writings from the Islamic world.
   • They used handbooks, called vademecums, and clinical observation to check their patients' conditions.
   • There were only about 100 physicians in England in 1300s and they were very expensive, so only the rich could afford them.

Apothecary:
   • Apothecaries treated their patients with remedies and gave advice on how to use them.
   • They were trained through apprenticeships.
   • Most apothecaries were men, but some were 'wise women' who sold herbal remedies.
   • They were the most accessible and common form of treatment in medieval England.

Barber-Surgeon:
   • Barber-surgeons performed minor surgical procedures.
   • They had little training.
   • They also cut people's hair.

2 Apothecaries were trained through apprenticeships, whereas quacks had no medical knowledge. It was dangerous to visit a quack because their remedies often did more harm than good.

3 a) Barber-surgeon — A hernia operation was a minor procedure often performed by barber-surgeons. A poor person wouldn't be rich enough to see a university-trained surgeon.

   b) Physician — They were very expensive, so only the rich could afford to see them. Rich people would choose to see a physician because they were well trained.

   c) Hospital — The main purpose of hospitals was to care for the sick and elderly. A monastic hospital would be able to provide food, water and a warm place to stay for a sick, elderly person with no family to help them.

   d) Apothecary / Quack — Apothecaries and quacks sold remedies, which would be suitable for someone with just a cough. A poor person wouldn't be able to afford a physician.

Thinking Historically

1 a) Evidence for — There were healthcare options available for every person. Poor people could get treatment from apothecaries, quacks or hospitals.
   Evidence against — Not all healthcare options were available to everyone, for example, trained physicians were only an option for the rich.

   b) Evidence for — Hospitals were more hygienic than most places, for example they separated clean and dirty water and had good systems for getting rid of sewage. This would have been beneficial for patients' health.
   Evidence against — Medieval hospitals provided food, water and warmth, but they didn't treat disease. There also weren't many hospitals in medieval England, so this limited their impact.

   c) Evidence for — Barber-surgeons had little training, so they might not perform surgery well or safely.
   Evidence against — Surgery was generally dangerous in the medieval period because there was no way to prevent blood loss, infection or pain.

2 a) Physicians had a lack of practical training. Practising on real patients would have helped them learn new methods of treatment on the job but only the rich could afford them. Their lack of practical training meant they were less able to discover new treatments or make progress in medicine.

   b) Apothecaries made and sold herbal remedies. Some of these remedies were written down in books called 'Herbals'. The fact that apothecaries used the same 'recipes' for making their remedies suggests that they weren't trying to progress medicine by attempting new remedies, but were just doing what other apothecaries had done before them.

Answers

c) Barber-surgeons' lack of training meant they didn't have the ability or desire to experiment with new treatments. As a result, there was not much progress made in surgery in medieval England.

Page 15 — Case Study: The Black Death
Knowledge and Understanding
1 a) • Bubonic plague was spread by the bites of fleas from rats on ships.
   • Symptoms included headaches, high temperatures and pus-filled swellings on the skin.
  b) • Pneumonic plague was spread by coughs and sneezes.
   • Infected people would find it painful to breath and would cough up blood.
2 The Black Death arrived in Britain in 1348. It resulted in a huge decrease in population — it killed at least a third of British people between 1348 and 1350.

Thinking Historically
1 a) • In 1349, Edward III ordered the Lord Mayor of London to clean filth from the city streets and remove bad smells to avoid 'bad air'.
   • Edward III closed Parliament in January 1349.
  b) • People fasted and prayed because they thought the Black Death was a punishment from God for sinful behaviour.
   • Believers in astrology carried diamonds, rubies and charms. Some people also used 'magic' potions to protect themselves.
   • People who believed that the plague was caused by an imbalance of the humours used purging and bloodletting.
   • Those who believed in the miasma theory carried strong smelling herbs and lit fires to 'purify' the air.
  c) • People in Winchester forced the bishop to build new cemeteries outside the town because they believed that being close to the bodies of dead victims could spread the plague.
   • The people of Gloucester stopped people from entering or leaving the town. This suggested that they believed the plague was spread by human contact.
2 a) The Church's belief that the Black Death was a punishment from God encouraged ineffective treatments, such as prayer and fasting. This belief discouraged people from looking for practical solutions for treating the plague because they thought it was God's will.
  b) People didn't have the scientific knowledge to find out what was causing the Black Death, so they were only able to base treatments on existing theories, like the Four Humours Theory and the miasma theory. These treatments were ineffective because the theories were incorrect.
  c) Belief in astrology encouraged ineffective practices to prevent the Black Death, such as carrying rubies and diamonds. This did nothing to stop the disease from spreading.
3 Medieval people were powerless to stop the Black Death because they didn't have the medical knowledge to understand its cause. Many of the treatments carried out at the time suggest they didn't realise the disease was spread by flea bites, coughs and sneezes. Instead, the treatments they used suggest they believed in other causes, such as punishment from God or an imbalance of humours. Without the knowledge or tools to discover the real cause of the disease, medieval people had no way of being able to stop the Black Death.

Page 17 — Exam-Style Questions
1 This question is level marked. You should look at the level descriptions on page 85 to help you mark your answer. Here are some points your answer may include:
   • There were less than 100 trained physicians in 1300. Although they had a better understanding of medicine than most medical healers, they lacked practical experience. Because there were only a few trained physicians and they had little practical experience, this meant that progress was slow and their treatments were often ineffective.
   • People often bought fake medicines from quacks who had no medical knowledge. Although these medicines were affordable, they often did more harm than good. The fact that these forms of medicine were affordable often made them the most accessible remedies for ordinary people, who couldn't afford to try new and more practical solutions.
   • Incorrect ideas about medicine were encouraged by the Roman Catholic Church. The Church was very influential, so people didn't look for new treatments that went against the Church's teachings. Instead, they continued using ineffective treatments promoted by the Church, such as prayer and repentance.
   • Science and technology weren't very advanced, meaning it was hard to discover new treatments. As a result, doctors relied on existing incorrect theories. For example, bloodletting continued to be used as a treatment by doctors because of their belief in the Four Humours theory, despite it doing more harm than good.
   • Dissection was outlawed by the Church. This meant people couldn't study the anatomy of the human body and therefore weren't able to develop their understanding of how it worked. Instead they continued to rely on Galen's incorrect teachings, which led to treatments based on inaccurate information.
2 This question is level marked. You should look at the level descriptions on page 85 to help you mark your answer. Here are some points your answer may include:
   • The Roman Catholic Church encouraged people to believe that disease was a punishment from God. Sick people would pray to be cured and some people would fast or go on pilgrimages. Because people believed that God caused disease, people's understanding of medicine didn't progress beyond theories that the Church promoted.
   • The Roman Catholic Church encouraged people to follow the ideas of ancient thinkers like Galen and Hippocrates without questioning them. Their theories about the causes of disease, such as the Theory of the Four Humours and the miasma theory, were incorrect. This meant that little progress was made in understanding the real causes of disease.
   • The Roman Catholic Church prevented doctors from dissecting human bodies. This meant doctors had to follow Galen's ideas about human anatomy. However, Galen had only ever dissected animals, so many of his ideas were based on incorrect assumptions about the human body. Because medieval doctors were unable to dissect human bodies, they weren't able to work out that Galen was wrong. Because they weren't disproved, Galen's incorrect ideas were assumed to be correct for a long time.

Answers

- Many medical healers in medieval England were poorly trained, and didn't have the knowledge or desire to investigate the causes of disease or find better treatments. For example, barber-surgeons' lack of training meant they didn't have the ability or the motivation to try new treatments. This contributed to the lack of development in medieval surgery.
- Medieval doctors ignored evidence which suggested that popular medical treatments were ineffective. For example, bloodletting often killed patients, but doctors continued to use this treatment. This reluctance to reject ineffective treatments meant that doctors didn't try to find alternative cures.

3 This question is level marked. You should look at the level descriptions on page 85 to help you mark your answer. Here are some points your answer may include:
- The Theory of the Four Humours was a rational explanation that severely limited medical progress because it was incorrect but still widely followed. It suggested that disease was caused by imbalances of four fluids in the body, which was later proved to be wrong. However, during the medieval period, the Roman Catholic Church supported this theory and the Church's great influence meant the theory was rarely challenged. This meant that people were less likely to consider other explanations for the causes of disease.
- The miasma theory was a rational explanation for disease, but it also limited medical progress because many people believed it even though it was incorrect. The miasma theory encouraged people to do hygienic things, like cleaning the streets, which helped to stop the spread of disease. Even though the miasma theory was wrong, this was used as evidence that it worked, which meant that many people believed it was correct. Because the miasma theory was so widely believed, people didn't challenge it until the 1860s.
- Rational explanations hindered medical progress because doctors ignored evidence that some treatments based on rational causes didn't work. For example, doctors still used bloodletting, based on the rational Theory of the Four Humours, even though it led to people dying. This meant that doctors continued to use ineffective treatments based on rational explanations rather than looking for alternative explanations.
- Supernatural theories about the causes of disease limited medical progress because they suggested humans were powerless to stop disease. Disease was often seen as a punishment from God in the medieval period. This meant people thought there was no practical way to prevent or treat disease, which meant they didn't understand the benefit of medical training or research.
- Some people believed that disease was caused by the movements of the planets and the stars. Doctors used almanacs to diagnose patients, which made their conclusions seem more reliable. This meant that people who believed in astrological causes of disease might not look for more rational explanations.

c.1500-c.1700: The Medical Renaissance in England

Page 19 — The Renaissance
Knowledge and Understanding
1 During the medieval period, people thought that disease was caused by an imbalance in the humours. The Four Humours Theory was also popular during the Renaissance period, thanks to the rediscovery of the original writings of Greek and Roman physicians like Hippocrates and Galen.
2 The invention of new weapons, such as cannons and guns, meant that doctors and surgeons had to find treatments for new injuries.
3 a) A Persian physician who lived from 980 to 1037 AD.
  b) A training college for doctors set up in 1518.
  c) An ingredient discovered by explorers that was believed to cure syphilis.
  d) A drug used to treat malaria, extracted from the bark of the Cinchona tree.
  e) The closing down of Britain's monasteries by Henry VIII in the 1530s.
  f) A device used to help with childbirth that was invented in the 1600s by Peter Chamberlen.

Thinking Historically
1 a) • Western doctors became more interested in the Four Humours Theory and treatment by opposites.
  • There was a greater focus on anatomy and dissection in medicine because many of the new books claimed that they were important. This encouraged people to reach their own conclusions about the causes of disease.
  • People began to question ancient doctors like Galen, although Galen's writings were still studied.
  b) • The Catholic Church had less control over medical teaching.
  • Hospitals that had been run by monasteries were closed down. This had a negative effect on people's health.
  • Monastic hospitals were slowly replaced by free hospitals. These were funded by charities and run by trained physicians who focused more on helping people to recover from illness.
  c) • Dissections became a key part of medical training for doctors who trained at the College of Physicians.
  • The licensing of doctors was encouraged to stop the influence of quacks, who sold fake medicines.
  • Some of the doctors who trained at the College of Physicians made important discoveries about disease and the human body, such as Harvey and his discoveries about the circulation of blood.
2 You can choose any option, as long as you explain your answer. For example:
The most important cause of change in medicine during the Renaissance period was attitudes in society. The reduced influence of the Church on medicine and the rediscovery of ancient books meant that people started to use dissection, direct observation and experimentation to learn how the body worked. This led to change in medicine, because it allowed doctors to challenge the ideas of Galen and make their own discoveries.

Answers

3 • Institutions like the College of Physicians had an important impact on medicine in the Renaissance period. However, the College was only able to carry out research and improve physicians' training because of the changes in society's attitudes towards dissection and direct observation. The impact of institutions depended on the change in society's attitudes.
 • Although there were some scientific and technological developments in the Renaissance period, they only had an isolated impact on the development of medicine as a whole. For example, forceps helped with childbirth, but had little impact on other areas of medicine.

Page 21 — Vesalius and Sydenham
Knowledge and Understanding
1 a) • Vesalius — Performed dissections on criminals who had been executed.
 • Sydenham — Made detailed observations of his patients and kept accurate records of their symptoms.
 b) • Vesalius — Believed that successful surgery was only possible if doctors had a proper understanding of the human body. He pointed out some of Galen's mistakes and made discoveries about anatomy. For example, he showed that there were no holes in the septum of the heart.
 • Sydenham — Thought that practical experience was more important than theoretical knowledge. He realised that diseases could be classified like animals or plants, and showed that scarlet fever was different to measles. He also introduced new treatments, e.g. he used laudanum to relieve pain, used iron to treat anaemia and treated malaria with quinine.
 c) • Vesalius — 'Six Anatomical Pictures' (1538) and 'The Fabric of the Human Body' (1543).
 • Sydenham — 'Medical Observations' (1676).
 d) • Vesalius — He showed how important it was to dissect bodies to find out how the human body was structured. He also encouraged other doctors to question Galen.
 • Sydenham — He showed the importance of diagnosis, and his descriptions of medical conditions helped other doctors to diagnose them. His ideas were used to train new doctors for over 200 years.
2 Diagnosis focuses on using the symptoms of disease to work out what the disease is, whereas prognosis is about predicting what the disease will do next.

Thinking Historically
1 a) Dissection of human bodies became an important part of medical training and research.
 b) The change was due to shifting attitudes in society, as religion played a less important role in medicine. It was also due to the influence of Vesalius, who showed that dissection was important to understand the human body.
 c) The printing press meant that new ideas, such as Vesalius' theories, could be spread more quickly.
 d) The invention of the printing press was a technological development.
 e) Galen's teachings began to be questioned more frequently by doctors who carried out their own experiments.
 f) This change was due to shifting attitudes in society as a result of the discovery of ancient books. Vesalius also had an influence on this change, because he showed that some of Galen's ideas were wrong and encouraged other doctors to make their own discoveries.

2 You can choose either option, as long as you explain your answer. For example:
 • Sydenham deserved the name 'the English Hippocrates'. His ideas had a long-term impact on how doctors diagnosed and treated their patients, as did Hippocrates' Four Humours Theory.

Page 23 — Case Study: William Harvey
Knowledge and Understanding
1 Before William Harvey, people believed that there were two kinds of blood that flowed through separate systems of blood vessels. They believed that 'nutrition-carrying' blood was purple and flowed from the liver through the veins to the rest of the body where it was used up. It was thought that 'life-giving' blood, which was bright red, was produced in the lungs and flowed through the arteries to the body, where it was consumed in the same way.
2 Harvey came up with a new theory that there was only one system of blood vessels and one kind of blood. He argued that blood circulated around the body instead of being constantly formed and used up.
3 The invention of a new type of water pump around the time Harvey was born gave him a model to compare the human heart to, because they both worked in a similar way.

Thinking Historically
1 • Vesalius used dissection to study the human anatomy more closely. Harvey developed this work by using the dissection of both humans and animals to make new discoveries.
 • Vesalius started to develop an understanding of how the human body works and produced accurate diagrams of it. Harvey built on this by adding new information about how blood circulates around the body.
2 • Surgical techniques and medical treatments were still very basic in Harvey's lifetime. This meant that although people knew more about blood and the body due to Harvey's research, complicated medical procedures like blood transfusions were usually unsuccessful.
 • It took a long time for Harvey's theories to be accepted and for doctors to use them in the treatments. For example, many doctors still believed in the Four Humours Theory, so they continued to use bloodletting as a treatment for disease.
3 a) Harvey used dissections and direct observation of living animal hearts to carry out his research. This encouraged other doctors to use similar methods.
 b) Harvey's research helped doctors to understand anatomy better than they had before. He showed that blood wasn't continually formed and consumed, but circulated around the body.
 c) Harvey's work proved that Vesalius had been right about the importance of dissection. His discoveries proved to other doctors that the best way to find out about the human body was to study it directly.
4 You can choose any option, as long as you explain your answer. For example:
 • Vesalius had the biggest impact on medical understanding because he was one of the first doctors to use dissection to find out more about how the human body worked. His research into anatomy was very influential — his works were spread by the printing press so a lot of people read his ideas.

Answers

Page 25 — Transmission of Ideas
Knowledge and Understanding
1   In the Renaissance period, the Royal Society was the centre of research into new scientific theories and new technology. The society encouraged people to question existing ideas and discover things for themselves.

2 a) Ambroise Paré's books were translated into several languages and reprinted. They spread information and ideas about performing surgery and influenced other books about surgery.

b) 'Philosophical Transactions' was the scientific journal of the Royal Society. It allowed more people to read about ideas, discoveries and inventions linked to the work of the Royal Society.

c) 'Micrographia' was a study written by Robert Hooke and published by the Royal Society in 1665. It showed the first drawings of a flea that had been made using a microscope.

3   The printing press encouraged people to question Galen's ideas because many different versions of Galen's books were printed. As a result, his writings seemed less reliable, because it wasn't clear what he had originally written.

Thinking Historically
1 a) • Students in universities could have their own textbooks because books could be copied much more easily. This meant that they could study in detail when they were training to be doctors.
  • New ideas about medicine could be spread and debated more easily. Before the printing press, texts had to be written by hand, so only widely accepted ideas were copied.
  • People began to question Galen's ideas because so many different versions of his old texts were printed.

b) • New scientific ideas were spread more easily due to the society's focus on sharing ideas and publishing its journal 'Philosophical Transactions'.
  • People were encouraged to question existing scientific ideas and make their own discoveries. The motto of the Royal Society translates as 'take no-one's word for it'.
  • People were exposed to new scientific theories and encouraged to trust new technology to help medicine progress.

2 a) The printing press and the Royal Society both had a great impact on society's attitudes to medicine. The invention of the printing press meant that new scientific ideas could be spread much more easily, which caused people to debate new medical ideas and question existing ones. The writings of Galen were questioned by an increasing number of people because so many different versions of his old books were printed, making it unclear what he had written originally. The Royal Society also promoted this questioning attitude by spreading new ideas through its scientific journal and encouraging people to be sceptical of existing ideas.

b) The printing press and the Royal Society both changed how medicine was studied, but they only had a limited impact on society's attitudes towards medicine. Most people in society couldn't read or write, so they were unaffected by the invention of the printing press or the discoveries of the Royal Society. Instead, the majority of people in this period still believed in medieval ideas about the causes of and treatments for disease.

c) Overall, I disagree that the printing press and the Royal Society transformed society's attitudes to medicine, because they only had an impact on a small section of society. Both the printing press and the Royal Society had a great impact on how medicine was studied and researched by doctors and scientists, but these changes had little impact on society as a whole because most people couldn't read or write.

3 a) Vesalius, Thomas Sydenham, William Harvey, Peter Chamberlen, Ambroise Paré, Robert Hooke

b) The Royal Society, the College of Physicians, free hospitals

c) The printing press, the development of new weapons, forceps, the water pump, the microscope, new ingredients for drugs

d) The Church had less influence on medicine, people began to believe in the importance of dissection, some people started to question the ideas of Galen and other ancient thinkers, there was more emphasis on direct observation and experimentation

4   You can choose any option, as long as you explain your answer. For example:
  • The work of individuals led to important developments. Once dissection was allowed, Vesalius and William Harvey made big breakthroughs in understanding the anatomy of the human body. Although their work didn't have an immediate impact on diagnosis and treatment, it provided an essential first step to improving them.

Page 27 — Medical Treatment: Continuity
Knowledge and Understanding
1   During the Renaissance period, people thought that the King's touch could cure scrofula. Thousands of people with scrofula visited Charles I so he could cure them.

2   • Apothecaries — They sold medicines in shops.
  • Barber-surgeons — They performed small operations.
  • Quack doctors — They sold medicines, although many of them were fake.

3   • Patients in hospitals were often made to work as well as being treated.
  • People with incurable or infectious diseases were often not allowed in hospitals.
  • People would visit hospitals to watch patients who were mentally disabled as a form of entertainment.
  • Many hospitals prioritised moral and spiritual education over improving the health of patients.

Thinking Historically
1   • Doctors were reluctant to accept that old ideas were wrong and were suspicious of new ideas.
  • Most people couldn't afford to see a doctor so they used other less-qualified healers.
  • Developments like the printing press and the Royal Society only affected a small number of people who could read.

2   Examples of continuity:
  • The ideas of ancient thinkers like Galen were still widely studied and often believed.
  • Doctors continued to use bloodletting as a treatment, even after William Harvey showed that the reasoning behind it was wrong.
  • Surgical techniques were still very basic, so complex surgery and blood transfusions remained dangerous.
  • Most people still couldn't read or write, so they were unaffected by developments like the printing press and the Royal Society.

92

Answers

- Most people still couldn't afford to visit trained doctors, so they relied on quacks, apothecaries and barber-surgeons.
- Superstition and religion still influenced people's ideas about the causes and treatments of disease.
- Most medical care still took place at home. People relied on wise women's herbal remedies and medical recipes passed down in the family.
- Hospital treatment remained basic and still wasn't accessible to everyone.

Examples of change:

- There was a rediscovery of ancient texts that encouraged people to question the ideas of Galen.
- The spread of Protestant Christianity reduced the influence of the Church in medicine, allowing people to question existing ideas more.
- Dissection became an important part of medical training thanks to the work of individuals like Vesalius and William Harvey, and training institutions like the College of Physicians.
- There were various advances in technology, such as the forceps, the microscope and new weapons that caused new kinds of injuries.
- New ingredients for medicines were discovered abroad. Some of these were used by doctors like Thomas Sydenham to develop new treatments.
- Free hospitals were set up to replace monastic hospitals — they were run by trained physicians and focused more on helping patients to get better. New hospitals like St Bartholomew's became centres of research.
- People like Vesalius and William Harvey made important discoveries about anatomy and blood circulation that helped to disprove Galen's theories and encourage other people to use dissection to find out more.
- The printing press meant that new ideas could be spread more quickly and people began to question the ideas of ancient thinkers.
- The Royal Society encouraged people to question existing ideas and make scientific discoveries for themselves.

3 You can answer either way, as long as you explain your answer. For example:

Overall, there was more change than continuity in the Renaissance period. For example, there was a significant move away from the theories of Galen and other ancient thinkers towards the use of direct observation and dissection to make medical discoveries. This shift was supported by the work of individuals like Vesalius, Sydenham and Harvey, as well as institutions like the Royal Society, and advances in technology like the printing press. Although these changes didn't affect everyone in society immediately, they changed people's understanding of how the human body worked and laid the foundations for future developments in medicine.

Page 29 — Case Study: The Great Plague

Knowledge and Understanding

1 The Great Fire of London burned down lots of the old, crowded houses. This may have killed plague bacteria and sterilised large parts of London.

2 The Great Plague killed about 100,000 people in London.

3 a) Carrying herbs and flowers to try to get rid of 'bad air'.
  b) Bloodletting
  c) Responses based on religion, such as praying and fasting.

Answers

4
- Councils tried to quarantine plague victims by locking them in their houses and painting a red cross and the words "Lord have mercy upon us" on their doors.
- Local councils organised carts to travel around the city collecting dead bodies for burial. They would then be buried in mass graves away from houses.
- Councils killed lots of dogs and cats because they thought that they were spreading the plague.

Thinking Historically

1 The plague had such a devastating impact on London because people didn't understand what caused the disease. Widespread beliefs like the miasma theory, the Theory of the Four Humours and superstition were wrong, so the methods of prevention and treatment based on them were usually ineffective. Official responses failed to limit the spread of the disease. There was no national government response, and measures introduced by local councils were largely ineffective because of the lack of understanding of what caused the disease. In addition, living conditions in London during the Renaissance were very bad — overcrowding and poverty made the Great Plague more deadly.

2
- In both cases, some people thought that the disease was a punishment from God, so they tried to prevent the spread of disease through prayer and fasting.
- People used bloodletting and purging as a treatment during both the Black Death and the Great Plague, due to their belief in the Four Humours Theory.
- During both outbreaks, people who believed in the miasma theory tried to 'purify' the air with herbs and flowers.
- People carried lucky charms, amulets and gemstones during both outbreaks due to their superstitious beliefs.
- During both outbreaks, attempts were made to stop the spread of the plague by preventing contact between healthy people and those with the disease. During the Black Death, Gloucester tried to avoid the plague by shutting itself off from the outside world, while local councils locked victims in their homes during the Great Plague.
- In both cases, people tried to distance themselves from the dead bodies of victims to stop the disease from spreading. In Winchester during the Black Death, the local people insisted that dead bodies be buried outside of the town. During the Great Plague, bodies were buried away from houses.
- There was no national government response to the outbreak of disease in both cases.

3 Even though there had been some progress in medicine between the two plague outbreaks, the causes of the plague and how it spread were no better understood in 1665 than they had been in the 14th century. As a result, the same ineffective responses were used during the Great Plague as during the Black Death.

Page 31 — Exam-Style Questions

1 This question is level marked. You should look at the level descriptions on page 85 to help you mark your answer. Here are some points your answer may include:

- Religion influenced attempts to prevent the spread of both the Black Death and the Great Plague. Both epidemics were believed by many to be a punishment from God for people's sins. Therefore, in both periods, people prayed in an attempt to prevent the spread of the disease.

Answers

- During both the Black Death and the Great Plague, there were attempts to prevent the disease from spreading by isolating people. During the Black Death, the people of Gloucester attempted to avoid the plague by shutting themselves off from the outside world. When the Great Plague hit London in 1665, councils tried to isolate plague victims by locking them in their houses and painting a red cross on their door.
- During both epidemics, people tried to prevent the spread of the disease by burying the dead away from places where people lived. When the Black Death reached Winchester, the local people insisted that new cemeteries be built outside the town rather than in the town centre. Similarly, during the Great Plague, the bodies of victims were buried in mass graves away from houses.

2   This question is level marked. You should look at the level descriptions on page 85 to help you mark your answer. Here are some points your answer may include:
- Vesalius improved people's knowledge and understanding of the human body. He drew accurate diagrams of the human body and was the first to show that there were no holes in the septum of the heart.
- Harvey's work advanced knowledge of circulation. People originally thought that there were two kinds of blood, which were created and consumed. Harvey showed that there was only one kind of blood, which circulated around the body.
- Dissections became a key part of medical training, allowing doctors to see inside the body for the first time. The work of Vesalius and Harvey showed the importance of dissection to developing new ideas about the human body.
- The printing press allowed individuals who made important discoveries about the human body to share them with others. For example, Vesalius published books of diagrams of the human body, such as 'The Fabric of the Human Body' (1543). The printing press allowed such books to be read by a larger audience.
- The Royal Society helped to spread new scientific theories, including new ideas about the human body. Its journal, 'Philosophical Transactions', allowed more people to read about these new ideas.
- Doctors began to challenge Galen for the first time, and this allowed new ideas about the human body to develop. In the Renaissance period, ancient texts were rediscovered which encouraged observation. This led to doctors examining the human body for themselves rather than relying on Galen. Vesalius and Harvey showed that Galen was wrong about how the human body worked, which encouraged others to question Galen. The declining influence of the Catholic Church, which had promoted Galen's ideas, also made it easier for doctors to challenge Galen.

3   This question is level marked. You should look at the level descriptions on page 85 to help you mark your answer. Here are some points your answer may include:
- Vesalius and Harvey offered alternative ideas about the human body. Vesalius drew accurate diagrams of the human body, while Harvey showed that blood circulates around the body.

- Ancient books discovered in the Renaissance period showed the value of observation and dissection. This encouraged doctors to learn by examining the body rather than relying on the theories of ancient doctors. This was an important first step in transforming doctors' beliefs about medicine.
- The rise of Protestant Christianity in Europe reduced the influence of the Catholic Church over medical teaching. This gave doctors more opportunity to challenge medical beliefs that had been promoted by the Catholic Church, such as Galen's teachings and supernatural beliefs about the causes of disease.
- Thomas Sydenham improved doctors' medical knowledge and altered their understanding of disease by introducing a new method of classifying diseases. This helped to change doctors' ideas about how they should treat their patients. Instead of focusing on prognosis, Sydenham encouraged doctors to examine patients' symptoms.
- The printing press allowed new ideas to spread more quickly. Doctors and university students could learn about new ideas from printed books. This encouraged them to try new theories and adopt new beliefs about medicine.
- The Royal Society encouraged people to question existing medical ideas. Its journal helped to spread new beliefs about medicine.
- Many people couldn't read, so new ideas in print didn't reach them. As a result, Galen's ideas about the causes and treatment of disease remained popular. Bloodletting was a common treatment during the Renaissance, even though Harvey had shown that it was based on a mistaken belief.
- Religious beliefs and the miasma theory remained popular in the Renaissance period. During the Great Plague, people used prayer, amulets and herbs (to 'purify' the air) to prevent the disease. This shows that, despite the new discoveries in the Renaissance period, many people did not alter their beliefs about medicine.

c.1700-c.1900: Medicine in 18th and 19th Century Britain

Page 33 — Case Study: Vaccination

Knowledge and Understanding

1   Smallpox was originally prevented through a process called inoculation. A cut was made in a patient's arm and then soaked in pus, which was taken from the swelling of somebody who already had a mild form of smallpox.

2   It didn't involve infecting the patient with smallpox, which could sometimes be deadly.

3
- 1796 — Jenner infected James Phipps with cowpox pus from the sores of Sarah Nelmes. He then infected Phipps with smallpox and Phipps didn't catch the disease.
- 1798 — Jenner published his findings about his vaccination.
- 1802 — Parliament approved of Jenner's vaccination and gave him £10,000 to open a clinic.
- 1840 — The smallpox vaccination was made free for infants.
- 1853 — The vaccination was made compulsory.

4   A laissez-faire style of government is when the government doesn't get involved with people's lives, including issues around healthcare.

Thinking Historically

1   • Doctors who gave the old smallpox inoculation thought they'd lose out financially — they saw Jenner's vaccination as a threat to their livelihood.
     • Lots of people were worried about giving themselves a disease from cows.

2 a) • Approved of Jenner's discovery and gave him £10,000 to open a clinic.
     • They gave Jenner a further £20,000.
     • They made the vaccination compulsory in 1853.

   b) • Lady Mary Wortley Montagu brought the method of inoculation from Turkey to Britain, which showed that smallpox could be prevented.
     • Edward Jenner discovered the link between smallpox and cowpox which led to the discovery of the vaccine.
     • James Phipps tested the first smallpox vaccination.
     • Sarah Nelmes' cowpox pus was used to infect James Phipps.

3   You can choose either option, as long as you explain your answer. For example:
     • Parliament was more important to the success of the smallpox vaccine. Initially, there was public opposition to Jenner's vaccination. However, once Parliament approved Jenner's research, this opposition faded. Parliament also funded a vaccination clinic and gave Jenner a further £20,000 a few years later. Without Parliament's support, Jenner's vaccination would not have reached as many people as it did, and wouldn't have been a success.

Page 35 — The Germ Theory

Knowledge and Understanding

1 a) The belief that germs were created by decaying matter, such as human waster or rotting food. It made people think that disease caused germs.

   b) The theory that microbes in the air caused decay and that some germs caused disease.

2   Pasteur showed that sterilised water that was kept in a closed flask stayed sterile, whereas sterilised water in an open flask bred germs. This suggested that there were germs in the air which entered the open flask.

3 a) anthrax spores
   b) the bacteria that cause septicaemia
   c) the bacteria that cause tuberculosis
   d) the bacteria that cause cholera

4   • agar jelly to create solid cultures and breed bacteria
     • dyes to stain bacteria so they were more visible under the microscope
     • photography to record his findings
     • advanced microscopes that allowed clearer images of small objects

Thinking Historically

1   People in both periods believed in the miasma theory, which suggested that 'bad air' caused disease.

2 a) It correctly explained how disease was caused, which allowed scientists to find effective treatments to disease.

   b) It showed that diseases could be prevented using vaccinations, which led to vaccinations being created for other diseases.

3   You can choose either option, as long as you explain your answer. For example:
     • The smallpox vaccine had a greater effect on the prevention of disease. Prior to the 1800s, doctors focused on finding cures for diseases, whereas Jenner's vaccination showed that prevention was an effective way to tackle disease. His work showed that vaccinations were safe, and this paved the way for more research into vaccinations and disease prevention.
     • The Germ Theory had a greater effect on the prevention of disease. It completely changed people's understanding of what caused disease and encouraged the government to introduce laws like the 1875 Public Health Act which helped stop diseases from spreading by improving living conditions. Pasteur's theory was also important for the discoveries of other scientists like John Snow, who used the theory to prevent cholera outbreaks.

Page 37 — Developments in Nursing

Knowledge and Understanding

1   Florence Nightingale studied to become a nurse in 1849, despite opposition from her family. After the Crimean War began, family friend and Secretary of War, Sidney Herbert asked Nightingale to go to Scutari to improve the nursing care at the Barrack Hospital.

2   Jamaica:
     • She learnt nursing from her mother, who ran a boarding house for soldiers.
     England (1854):
     • She came to volunteer as a nurse in the Crimean War, but was rejected, possibly for racial reasons.
     • Despite this rejection, she paid her own way to Crimea.
     Crimea:
     • She sold goods to travellers and soldiers while nursing soldiers back to health on the battlefield.
     • She built the British Hotel, a group of makeshift buildings that were used as a hospital, shop and soldier canteen.
     England (After the Crimean War):
     • After returning from the War, she went bankrupt because she couldn't find work as a nurse. However, she received some support due to press interest.

Thinking Historically

1   Nightingale changed nursing by emphasising the importance of hygiene. She published her teachings in 'Notes on Nursing' in 1859, which became the standard textbook for generations of nurses. Nightingale also changed the training received by nurses when she set up the Nightingale School of Nursing, which provided nurses with three years of training. During her lifetime, Nightingale also changed the reputation of nursing, making it a better respected profession.

2 a) • Medieval hospitals — there were relatively few.
     • Hospitals in 19th century — many more were built in this period.

   b) • Medieval hospitals — run by monasteries.

   c) • Medieval hospitals — provided sick and elderly people with a warm place to stay as well as food and clean water.

   d) • Medieval hospitals — were hygienic. Waste was kept separate from clean water and they had a good sewage system.
     • Hospitals in 19th century — they became cleaner and more hygienic during this period.

Answers

3   You can choose any option, as long as you explain your answer. For example:
Hospitals weren't very similar in the two time periods. During the medieval period, hospitals provided the sick and elderly with a comfortable place to stay, whereas hospitals in the 19th century were more focused on treating illnesses. Also, hospitals in the medieval period were often run by monks, whereas 19th-century hospitals were run by local authorities.

4   The Germ Theory had a limited effect on Florence Nightingale because the theory was only published in 1861, seven years after she left Crimea. Nightingale believed in the miasma theory, so although her focus on good hygiene prevented germs from spreading, she had no real knowledge why that was the case.

Page 39 — Anaesthetics
Knowledge and Understanding
1   They stop patients feeling pain during surgery. This is important because patients can die from the trauma of extreme pain.
2   a) Professor of Midwifery who discovered the effects of chloroform in 1847.
b) British chemist who identified nitrous oxide (laughing gas) as a possible anaesthetic in 1799.
c) American doctor who discovered that ether could be used as an anaesthetic in 1842.
d) American dentist who used nitrous oxide in a public demonstration in 1845.
e) In 1884, he investigated the use of cocaine as a local anaesthetic.
f) American dental surgeon who carried out the first public demonstration of ether as an anaesthetic in 1846.
3   a) It doesn't work on everyone.
b) It's an irritant and is also fairly explosive.
c) It can sometimes affect a patient's heart, which can cause them to die suddenly.
d) It's addictive.
4   There was an increased death rate in surgeries during this period.

Thinking Historically
1   You can choose any person, so long as you explain your answer. For example:
Humphry Davy made the most important contribution by beginning the process of trying to find a suitable anaesthetic. Furthermore, of all the anaesthetics identified in the 18th and 19th centuries, nitrous oxide was the only one that didn't risk harming the patient.
2   Here are some points your answer may include:
Positive effect:
• Anaesthetics made patients easier to operate on, which meant surgeons didn't have to rush their procedures.
• Developments in anaesthetics meant that more complicated surgeries could be carried out.
Negative effect:
• Anaesthetics led to more complex surgeries, which caused increased death rates because surgeons were more ambitious.
• Anaesthetics caused longer operating times, which meant there was an increased death rate due to infection.

3   a) Continuity — surgeons still didn't know clean clothes could prevent infection, so they often wore the same dirty coats for years.
b) Change — different anaesthetics were being trialled that began to replace natural drugs like alcohol and opium as pain relief during surgery.
c) Continuity — surgeries continued to be carried out in unhygienic locations, such as people's homes.
d) Change — operations became longer because unconscious patients were easier to operate on, so surgeons didn't have to rush.

Page 41 — Antiseptics
Knowledge and Understanding
1   Antiseptic surgical methods aim to kill germs, whereas aseptic surgical methods aim to prevent germs from entering the operating theatre.
2   He showed doctors that they could wash their hands with chloride of lime to reduce the spread of infection.
3   a) Lister saw carbolic acid being used in sewage works to keep down the smell. He tried it in his operating theatre in the early 1860s and infection rates reduced.
b) Lister heard about the Germ Theory, and realised that he could apply carbolic acid to instruments and bandages to kill germs.
4   It was unpleasant to get on your skin or breathe in, so doctors and nurses didn't like using it.
5   • They have sterilised instruments with high temperature steam.
• They have sterilised their hands before entering the operating theatre.
• They have worn sterilised gowns, masks, gloves and hats.
• They have kept the theatres clean and filled them with sterile air.
6   • 1846-1870 — The 'Black Period' of surgery where there was an increased death rate.
• early 1860s — Carbolic acid is used in operating theatres and reduces infection rates.
• 1867-1870 — The use of antiseptics in surgery reduces the death rate to around 15%.
• 1889 — William Halsted invents surgical gloves.

Thinking Historically
1   Joseph Lister introduced antiseptics in operating theatres, which reduced infection and subsequently death rates. This made patients less fearful of surgery by making it safer.
2   • Made surgery more germ-free, which reduced the death rates from around 50% to 15%.
• Allowed surgeons to operate with less fear of patients dying from infection.
• The number of operations increased tenfold from 1867-1912.
3   You can choose either option, as long as you explain your answer. For example:
• Antiseptics had a greater effect on 19th-century surgery. Although anaesthetics had a positive impact on surgery, they also contributed to increased death rates due to a higher rate of infection as a result of longer surgeries. Antiseptics, however, decreased infection rates during surgery and made procedures safer.

Answers

Page 43 — Case Study: Cholera in London

Knowledge and Understanding

1   Cholera is a disease that is caused by infected sewage entering drinking water. It causes extreme diarrhoea, which can lead to death. It reached Britain in 1831 and caused four epidemics between 1832 and 1866. It killed tens of thousands of people in Britain during the 19th century.

2   John Snow believed that cholera was a waterborne disease, but could not prove it. When cholera broke out in Broad Street in 1854, he investigated where people who had the disease got their drinking water. He discovered that they all used the same water pump on Broad Street. He convinced the local council to remove the water pump handle, which ended the outbreak in that area.

3   a) • John Snow — He had a theory about the link between cholera and water, and used this theory to investigate a cholera outbreak. He interviewed people close to the outbreak and his findings supported his theory that cholera is a waterborne disease.
   • Edward Jenner — He had a theory about the link between smallpox and cowpox. He tested his theory by infecting Phipps with cowpox and then smallpox. After observing Phipps, he concluded that cowpox could be used to prevent smallpox.
   b) • John Snow — He published a report 'On the Mode of Communication of Cholera' in 1855.
   • Edward Jenner — He published his findings in 1798.
   c) • John Snow — The local council removed the handle from the water pump which was suspected of causing the cholera outbreak.
   • Edward Jenner — The government gave him £30,000 to fund his work, and they eventually made his vaccination compulsory.

Thinking Historically

1   a) Living conditions were cramped and dirty, and people shared outdoor toilets called privies which made it easy for diseases like cholera to spread.
   b) Lots of people moved to the city to find work, which meant that the population of cities increased. This meant that more people were susceptible to outbreaks.
   c) Household waste and waste from cesspits were thrown into rivers, which led to contaminated water supplies.
   d) Water supplies were shared by several houses and the water was often contaminated by waste. This increased the likelihood of a cholera outbreak.

2   Although John Snow's findings were only accepted after the Germ Theory was published, they helped to change attitudes to public health. People began to believe that it was the government's responsibility to clean the streets and ensure people had access to clean water in order to prevent diseases like cholera. This change in attitudes led to the government introducing the 1875 Public Health Act.

Page 45 — The Public Health Act, 1875

Knowledge and Understanding

1   He published a report suggesting that poor living conditions caused poor health. This led to the 1848 Public Health Act, which tried to improve living conditions and the health of people living in towns and cities.

2   The 1875 Public Health Act was compulsory, whereas the one in 1848 said that towns could set up a health board or spend money only if they wanted to.

3   a) Councils appointed health and sanitary inspectors who made sure laws on water supplies and hygiene were followed. It also made councils maintain sewerage systems and keep their town's streets clean.
   b) It allowed local councils to buy slums with poor living conditions and turn them into houses that were built to a government-approved standard.
   c) This stopped people dumping sewage and industrial waste into rivers, which stopped water becoming contaminated.

Thinking Historically

1   • The Germ Theory — it linked disease to poor living conditions, which could be changed by the government.
   • Jenner's development of the smallpox vaccination — the government's involvement was successful in treating smallpox.
   • Nightingale's development of nursing — showed how making hospitals more hygienic would reduce disease and demonstrated the importance of training nurses. This led the government to pass the Nurses Registration Act in 1919, making training compulsory for all nurses.
   • The Second Reform Act — this act gave an additional 1 million men the vote. Many of these men were industrial workers. This meant that the government became more involved in healthcare because they had to listen to the needs of working-class people.

2   Here are some points you may include:
   • Louis Pasteur's Germ Theory was more significant in preventing disease than the government. It proved numerous theories, such as Snow's discovery that cholera was waterborne, which forced the government to take action. Without the Germ Theory, the government wouldn't have been under pressure to create the 1875 Public Health Act, and as a result there wouldn't have been as great an improvement in disease prevention in this period.
   • The government backed scientific findings which prevented disease. After Jenner published his findings about the smallpox vaccination, the government approved his discovery and gave him £10,000 to open a vaccination clinic. The government's backing led to the success of Jenner's smallpox vaccination by making it available, and later compulsory, to the general public. This significantly aided the prevention of smallpox in Britain.
   • Improvements in technology were the most significant factor in improving the prevention of disease c.1700-c.1900. Many scientific breakthroughs, such as Pasteur's Germ Theory and Koch's work on microbes, came about partly due to improved microscopes. This technological advancement aided several important discoveries, and without it there would have been less progress in disease prevention during this time period.

Pages 46-47 — Exam-Style Questions

1   This question is level marked. You should look at the level descriptions on page 85 to help you mark your answer. Here are some points your answer may include:
   • Disease prevention in the Renaissance period was mainly based on religious and superstitious ideas. For example, during the Great Plague, people would say prayers or carrying charms to protect them from catching the disease. In contrast, doctors in the 19th century used scientific ideas to prevent disease. For example, after reading about the Germ Theory, Joseph Lister began using carbolic acid during surgery to prevent infection.

- During the Renaissance period, the government did very little to prevent disease. For example, during the Great Plague, there was no government response to prevent the disease from spreading, and the outbreak only ended in London after the Great Fire of London. However, during the period c.1700-c.1900, the government did more to prevent diseases from spreading. For example, the 1875 Public Health Act enforced the maintenance of sewerage systems in order to prevent outbreaks of cholera.

2 This question is level marked. You should look at the level descriptions on page 85 to help you mark your answer. Here are some points your answer may include:

- Joseph Lister's work in the development of antiseptics led to the use of carbolic acid in operating theatres. This reduced the number of deaths due to infection. His work also arguably led to research into aseptics, which improved surgery further.
- Anaesthetics were developed to stop patients feeling pain. The pain felt by patients during surgery was a severe problem, as it could lead to death by trauma. It also meant procedures had to be short, and performing surgery on conscious patients was also very difficult. James Simpson's experimentation with chloroform and its use by Queen Victoria during the birth of her eighth child led to it becoming a widely used anaesthetic.
- The publication of the Germ Theory meant that surgeons were aware that germs which caused disease could be airborne. This led to more surgeries being performed in aseptic environments, rather than in people's homes. This contributed to fewer deaths in surgery as a result of infection. The awareness that cleanliness was important for medical procedures improved surgery.
- The approach to tackling germs in surgery changed in the late 1800s from using antiseptics to kill germs to using asepsis to prevent germs. Aseptic methods included sterilising surgical instruments before use with steam, wearing clean, sterilised gowns and gloves, and sterilising the air in the theatre. These methods improved surgery because preventing germs in the first place reduced the chance of a patient getting infected.

3 This question is level marked. You should look at the level descriptions on page 85 to help you mark your answer. Here are some points your answer may include:

- In the Renaissance period, individuals like Vesalius and Harvey made important discoveries about human anatomy that advanced medical knowledge. However, the impact of these ideas on health and medicine relied on improvements in communication. Without developments like the introduction of the printing press in the 1470s, it is unlikely that individuals like Vesalius would have been able to spread their ideas as widely as they did.
- In the Renaissance period, changing attitudes helped to create the conditions for individuals' discoveries. For example, the decline of the Catholic Church's influence made it easier for individuals like Harvey and Vesalius to question Galen's teachings on the human body. Unlike earlier individuals, Vesalius could dissect corpses to examine Galen's ideas — the Church had previously prevented people from performing dissections on humans.

- The work of individuals was a very important factor in the development of health and medicine in the 18th and 19th centuries. In the late 18th century, Jenner developed the smallpox vaccine. In the 19th century, Pasteur and Koch made important discoveries about the causes and prevention of disease. The work of Simpson and Lister helped to make surgery safer in the 19th century. These individuals all helped to advance the development of health and medicine in Britain.
- In the 19th century, individuals were important in highlighting public health problems and campaigning for change. John Snow linked cholera to contaminated water. Nightingale campaigned for better hospital care. Chadwick played a role in the development of public health provision. However, it was the government's willingness to act on the concerns of these individuals that led to significant developments in health and medicine.
- Government funding was also an important factor in the development of health and medicine in the 19th century. In the early 19th century, the government paid a total of £30,000 to fund Jenner's work, which allowed him to open a vaccination clinic and prevent more people from getting smallpox.
- Technology also helped many individuals make their discoveries. Harvey's discoveries about the heart were inspired by a new water pump. Pasteur's Germ Theory was aided by the introduction of microscopes which allowed him to see germs more clearly.

4 This question is level marked. You should look at the level descriptions on page 85 to help you mark your answer. Here are some points your answer may include:

- Medieval beliefs about the causes of diseases were based on old ideas, whereas in the 19th century the ideas about the causes of diseases were based on new ideas and scientific experimentation. In medieval times, people believed that an imbalance of the Four Humours caused disease — this was based on the work of Hippocrates, an Ancient Greek physician. In the 1860s, Joseph Lister's use of antiseptics to prevent infection during surgery was based on Germ Theory, an idea that was published in 1861.
- A major difference between the two periods is the change in attitude towards the miasma theory. During the medieval period, people believed that breathing in 'bad air' caused diseases. However, Pasteur's publication of the Germ Theory in 1861 suggested that disease was caused by germs in the air. By the end of the 19th century, beliefs were beginning to shift away from the miasma theory as a cause of disease and towards the Germ Theory.
- During the medieval period, the Catholic Church was very influential in medicine. Medieval people believed that disease was caused by God as a punishment for sinful behaviour. However, by the period c.1700-c.1900, the Church had less influence over medicine, so scientists looked more closely at rational explanations for the causes of disease. For example, in 1855, John Snow believed that cholera was caused by contaminated water.

Answers

5   This question is level marked. You should look at the level descriptions on page 85 to help you mark your answer. Here are some points your answer may include:

• Prior to the 19th century, the government had a laissez-faire attitude to healthcare — they didn't think it was their responsibility to get involved with public health. However, by the 19th century, individuals were placing more pressure on the government to prevent disease. For example, John Snow's work on cholera led to the 1875 Public Health Act, which required local councils to properly maintain sewerage systems and prevent the contamination of drinking water. This prevented further cholera outbreaks.

• The work of Florence Nightingale helped to improve hospital sanitation which reduced the spread of disease and deaths from infection. Nightingale's book 'Notes on Nursing' emphasised the need for hygiene and well-trained nurses. By 1900, there were 64,000 nurses who were using Nightingale's techniques to prevent disease in hospitals.

• Before the 19th century, people didn't understand how diseases were caused — many still believed in the miasma theory. Pasteur's Germ Theory (1861) suggested that disease was caused by airborne germs, rather than just 'bad air'. This development allowed scientists to effectively prevent disease, for example, Joseph Lister used Germ Theory to introduce antiseptics to surgery to prevent infection.

• The government funded campaigns that aimed to prevent disease. In 1802, they gave Edward Jenner £10,000 to open a smallpox vaccination clinic in order to prevent the spread of the disease. This support, as well as making vaccination against smallpox compulsory in 1853, contributed to the vaccination's success and led to a large fall in the number of smallpox cases in Britain.

• Advancements in technology helped scientists make important breakthroughs. For example, improvements in microscope technology in the 1800s meant that Pasteur was able to view microbes more clearly. This led to the development of the Germ Theory — this was instrumental in preventing disease, as it influenced Lister's work on antiseptics and Snow's work on cholera.

6   This question is level marked. You should look at the level descriptions on page 85 to help you mark your answer. Here are some points your answer may include:

• The Germ Theory was an important breakthrough because it was the first time germs had been shown to cause disease. Before the Germ Theory, many people believed that disease was caused by miasma. This meant people did not know how to effectively prevent dangerous diseases like cholera.

• The Germ Theory proved previous discoveries to be correct, which led to important changes in social health. John Snow's discovery about cholera being linked to contaminated water wasn't widely accepted until the Germ Theory proved it to be true. Once it was proven true, institutions like the government were willing to act to improve hygiene in towns and cities based on Snow's findings.

• The Germ Theory showed that hygiene was important in preventing infection. This led to important improvements in surgery, such as Joseph Lister's use of antiseptic carbolic acid on instruments and bandages, and the development of aseptic surgery.

• The Germ Theory showed there was a link between poor living conditions and disease. This supported the findings of Edwin Chadwick and put pressure on the government to pass the 1875 Public Health Act.

• While the Germ Theory helped figures like Robert Koch link diseases to specific microbes, it was a long time before its full impact on the treatment of disease was felt. The first magic bullet was only developed in 1909. Penicillin, the first antibiotic, wasn't discovered until 1928.

• Many improvements to people's health in the 19th century took place before the discovery of the Germ Theory. Jenner's smallpox vaccine led to a big fall in the number of smallpox cases, even though people didn't know why it worked. Nightingale's improvements in hospital sanitation helped prevent deaths, even though she didn't know that germs caused disease.

c.1900-Present: Medicine in Modern Britain

Page 49 — Modern Ideas on the Causes of Disease

Knowledge and Understanding

1 a) Ivanovsky investigated a disease that was killing tobacco plants and found an extremely small microbe that remained in water even after bacteria were removed. This led to further findings by other scientists.

   b) Beijernick discovered that the microbes Ivanovsky found had different properties to bacteria. He called them viruses.

   c) Crick and Watson discovered that DNA can reproduce itself by splitting, describing it as a double helix. This allowed other scientists to find genes that caused genetic conditions.

2   A genetic condition is a disease that's caused by faulty genes and is passed on from one generation to another. Examples of genetic conditions include cystic fibrosis, haemophilia and sick-cell anaemia.

3   • Smoking — can cause lung cancer.
    • Obesity — increases the chance of heart disease or diabetes.
    • Too much alcohol — can cause liver disease.
    • Too much sunlight / sunburn — can lead to skin cancer.

Thinking Historically

1   You can choose either option, as long as you explain your answer. For example:

• The discovery of DNA had a bigger impact on modern medicine because it provided an explanation for previously unexplained illnesses, such as haemophilia, which are caused by faulty genes. This discovery led to the development of treatments for genetic diseases using techniques such as gene therapy. The discovery of DNA also proved that some diseases are inherited, which identified a new way for diseases to spread. Although the discovery of viruses was important, the body is able to destroy some viruses without treatment whereas genetic conditions need medical intervention to treat them.

Answers

2 Renaissance England (c.1500-c.1700):
- Punishment from God
- An imbalance of the Four Humours
- Bad air (the miasma theory)

c.1900-Present:
- Bacteria
- Viruses
- Genetic conditions
- Lifestyle factors

3 Here are some points your answer may include:
- Ideas around the causes of disease were different. Since c.1900, doctors are aware that there is more than one cause of disease, for example viruses and genetic conditions. However in Renaissance England, doctors had less knowledge about the causes of disease, and relied on applying the same incorrect causes, such as the miasma theory. This means that treatment and prevention of diseases has become far more complex since c.1900 than it was in Renaissance England.
- Ideas around the causes of disease were different because social attitudes in Renaissance England were different to social attitudes today. For example, during the Renaissance, religion and superstition influenced many people's ideas about the causes of disease, whereas the development of modern scientific methods from c.1900 means that those explanations are no longer widely accepted.
- I think ideas around the causes of disease were similar. Both periods used scientific reasoning of the time to inform their ideas about the causes of disease. For example, in the 1600s Thomas Sydenham observed his patients and kept detailed records. This is similar to the way that doctors today try to identify the causes of disease.

Page 51 — Developments in Diagnosis
Knowledge and Understanding
1
- 1880s/1890s — Blood pressure monitors are invented — these let doctors see whether disease, lifestyle factors or medicines are causing high blood pressure.
- 1895 — Wilhelm Röntgen discovers X-rays. These allow doctors to see what is happening inside a patient.
- Mid-20th century — Blood sugar monitors were developed to allow people with diabetes to make sure their blood sugar is at the right level.
- 1972 — Godfrey Hounsfield invents Computed Tomography (CT or CAT) scans. They use X-rays and a computer to make detailed images of parts of the patient's body.
- 1980s — Magnetic Resonance Imaging (MRI) scans become widely used. They construct images using powerful radio waves and magnetic fields.

2 In ultrasound scanning, high frequency sound waves are used to create an image of the inside of a patient's body. The sound waves bounce off a patient's organs or other tissues, creating an image of these organs on the computer.

Thinking Historically
1 a) Blood tests have made diagnosis more accurate — they give doctors clearer information of what is wrong with a patient. They also enable doctors to check cholesterol levels, to predict the chance of heart attack or stroke, as well as check for genetic conditions or whether a patient has a certain type of cancer.

b) X-rays allow doctors to see what is happening inside their patients' bodies. This means that doctors can establish the cause of disease earlier, which gives them a better chance of treating the disease successfully.

c) Blood pressure monitors allow doctors to see whether high blood pressure is being caused by disease, lifestyle factors or medicines. They can also be used by people in their own homes, giving patients the ability to monitor and improve their own health. This means that doctors and patients can monitor blood pressure before it leads to more serious problems.

2 You can choose any option, as long as you explain your answer. For example:
I think that blood tests have had the most significant impact on modern medicine. They allow doctors to diagnose a wide range of health issues, such as cancer and genetic conditions, and early diagnosis often leads to more successful treatment.

3 Methods of diagnosis weren't very similar between these periods. From 1900 onwards, doctors used technology to accurately diagnose the cause of disease, whereas doctors in medieval England used non-scientific methods to diagnose patients, such as astrology.

4 Here are some points your answer may include.
- Scientific discoveries were more important to the development of medicine. Crick and Watson's discovery of DNA in 1953 enabled doctors to identify and treat the faulty genes that cause disease. Prior to their discovery, genetic conditions, such as cystic fibrosis were difficult to treat, but their work has led to the development of gene therapy.
- New technology was more important to the development of medicine. The introduction of CT and MRI scans have given doctors a clearer picture of the inside of their patients' bodies. This means they can intervene much earlier, which leads to more effective treatments that have a higher chance of success.
- Overall, although scientific discoveries are vital to the development of medicine, they are only possible because of new technology. Therefore I disagree with the statement.

Page 53 — Case Study: Penicillin
Knowledge and Understanding
1 Penicillin is an antibiotic. It is important because it is used to treat a range of bacterial infections and its discovery led to the development of other antibiotic treatments.

2 Fleming was researching an antiseptic for staphylococcal bacteria. In 1928, he realised that a fungal spore had landed in one of his culture dishes by chance. The mould had stopped the colonies of staphylococcal from growing. The fungal spore, Penicillium notatum, produced a substance that killed bacteria and it was named penicillin.

3 No one was willing to fund further research, so Fleming was unable to develop the industrial production of penicillin.

4 Florey and Chain didn't have the resources to produce penicillin in large amounts. Even though their patient had begun to recover during the first clinical trial, Florey and Chain ran out of penicillin and the patient died.

Answers

Thinking Historically

1 a) Fleming wanted to find a cure for staphylococcal bacteria. This led to his discovery of penicillin.

   b) This meant that penicillin could be purified, which was important as penicillin couldn't be used in its natural state. This was crucial in preparing penicillin for industrial production.

   c) America gave out grants to businesses that manufactured penicillin. By 1943, British businesses were also mass-producing penicillin which meant military medics had sufficient amounts by 1944.

   d) This made penicillin more accessible for general use.

2 Institutions were significant in the success of penicillin. Funding from the American government led to the mass production of penicillin, which allowed penicillin to be distributed to military medics. Without involvement from the government and the companies which mass-produced penicillin, penicillin would not have been a success, because Fleming was unable to take his initial work further without funding from institutions.

3 You can choose either option, so long as you explain your answer. For example:
   • The discovery of penicillin had more of an impact on medicine than Jenner's work. Penicillin was the first antibiotic and it is still used to treat a range of bacterial infections. There was already an inoculation for smallpox when Jenner discovered his vaccination, meaning Jenner's work had less of an impact compared to the discovery of penicillin.

Page 55 — Modern Treatments

Knowledge and Understanding

1 A magic bullet is a synthetic antibody. They are called 'magic bullets' because they only attack specific microbes.

2 • 1889 — Ehrlich begins to research chemicals that could act as synthetic antibodies.
   • 1905 — The bacterium that causes syphilis is identified.
   • 1909 — Sahachiro Hata joins the team and rechecks the results. He notices that compound number 606 appeared to work.
   • 1911 — Salvarsan 606 is used for the first time under its trade name.

3 a) Radiotherapy — targeted X-rays and gamma rays are used to kill cancer cells — 1896-1898

   b) Chemotherapy — drugs are used to target cancer cells and reduce tumours — during World War II

   c) Targeted therapy — drugs that prevent cancer from spreading — late-20th century

Thinking Historically

1 The Germ Theory was the discovery that germs cause disease. This meant that scientists such as Ehrlich and Domagk knew that they had to study germs if they wanted to be able to treat disease. This influenced their research on antibodies — they knew that antibodies fought germs in the body, and they wouldn't have known this without the Germ Theory.

2 Here are some points your answer may include:
   Medieval England:
   • Bloodletting
   • Purging
   • Prayer/Repentance
   • Exorcisms
   • Lucky charms
   • Smelling herbs/burning incense
   • Herbal remedies

20th century:
   • Synthetic antibodies/magic bullets
   • radiotherapy
   • chemotherapy
   • targeted therapy
   • antibiotics/penicillin
   • antiviral drugs
   • changing lifestyle factors

3 Treatments in these two periods weren't similar. Treatments in the medieval period were ineffective due to a lack of technology and a limited understanding of the causes of disease. For example, bloodletting was a treatment which involved cutting the patient or applying leeches to remove excessive blood and 'rebalance' the Four Humours. However, patients regularly died from this treatment. In the 20th century, treatments were a lot more advanced, such as synthetic antibodies which target specific microbes within the body to cure disease. These treatments are more effective and much safer for the patient.

Page 57 — Modern Surgery

Knowledge and Understanding

1 Landsteiner discovered blood groups and found that blood transfusions could be carried out safely as long as the patient's blood group matched the blood donor's.

2 a) During World War I, doctors found that sodium citrate prevented blood from clotting. This meant that they could store it outside the body and set up blood banks so that transfusions could be performed, which helped to prevent excess blood loss during surgery.

   b) Immunosuppressants are important in organ transplants. They stop the immune system from attacking the implant, which makes organ transplants safer and increases their success rate.

3 Keyhole surgery is a less invasive type of surgery that is carried out using an endoscope inserted through a small cut.

Thinking Historically

1 You can choose any option, so long as you explain your answer. For example:
   Keyhole and robot-assisted surgery has had the biggest impact on modern medicine because it has made surgery safer. For example, using smaller cuts means there is reduced blood loss and it decreases the risk of infection.

2 Surgery in c.1700-c.1900:
   • More reliable anaesthetics used to numb pain during surgery.
   • Antiseptics introduced to kill germs and reduce the chance of infection.
   • Aseptic methods used to prevent germs entering the operating theatre.
   Surgery from 1900 onwards:
   • Blood transfusions during surgery are more successful.
   • Organ transplants carried out successfully.
   • Keyhole and robot-assisted surgery has made surgery safer.

Answers

3   You can choose either option, so long as you explain your answer. For example:
There was a greater change in surgery during c.1700-c.1900. Surgery was considered unsafe prior to c.1700, with many patients dying due to infection and trauma. The introduction of antiseptics and anaesthetics led to a drop in death rates and made surgery much safer which meant the number of surgeries increased. Although there have been improvements in surgery from c.1900 onwards, this progress might not have happened without the changes that were made in c.1700-c.1900.

4   Barber-surgeons:
   • Had little to no knowledge or training
   • Had no desire to improve surgery
   • Weren't very well respected
   • Also cut hair
   • Only performed basic surgeries
   Modern surgeons:
   • Trained at university and medical school
   • Have attempted to develop surgical procedures, such as Christiaan Barnard who carried out the first successful heart transplant.
   • Highly-respected profession
   • Perform complex surgeries

Page 59 — The National Health Service

Knowledge and Understanding

1 a) Number of infant deaths, showing the risk of childbirth before the NHS — 1901
   b) Percentage of physically unfit volunteers for military service during the Boer War — 1899
   c) Percentage of doctors who initially joined the NHS — 1948
   d) Number of doctors in Britain — between 1948 and 1973

2 a) Beveridge contributed to the changing social attitudes towards healthcare. He published a report which demanded the government do more for healthcare. When the Labour Party was elected in 1945 they implemented Beveridge's proposals by founding the NHS.
   b) Bevan introduced the NHS when he was the Minister of Health. He wanted the NHS to be free for patients so he introduced a system of National Insurance to pay for it. He convinced doctors and dentists to work for the NHS by giving them a payment for each patient they registered, while allowing them to continue treating private patients. This led to 92% of doctors and all hospitals joining the NHS.

Thinking Historically

1   Renaissance Period:
   • Ordinary people couldn't afford to be treated by trained physicians.
   • They bought medicines from quacks or from apothecaries.
   • Treated at home/cared for by family members.
   • Unhygienic living conditions and overcrowding often meant that the poor were hit worst by disease.
   Early 20th century:
   • The health of the general public was generally poor — 40% of volunteers were physically unfit for military service.
   • Access to healthcare was limited as a lot of poor people couldn't afford to go to the doctor.
   • Many ordinary people couldn't afford to buy medicine.

2   Health and healthcare for ordinary people were similar during these periods. Access to the best healthcare in both periods was expensive so poor people couldn't afford it. Ordinary people were also generally unhealthy in both periods.

3   World War I:
   • Fleming witnessed soldiers die of septic wounds which inspired him to conduct research that led to the discovery of penicillin.
   • Surgeons developed techniques for skin transplantations.
   • The war drained Britain's resources, which contributed to the government being unable to expand healthcare provisions in the 1920s and 1930s.
   World War II:
   • Nitrogen mustard, a chemical in mustard gas, was discovered by doctors. Its discovery led to the use of chemotherapy to treat cancer.
   • The war led to a change in public attitudes towards healthcare. The raising of a mass army made people realise the health problems of the poor.
   • The government set up the Emergency Medical Service to treat air raid casualties. This proved that centralised control of medical services could be successful.

4   You can choose any option, so long as you explain your answer. For example:
The work of individuals was the main reason the NHS was created, rather than World War II. While World War II made people aware of the health issues surrounding soldiers from poor backgrounds, this had also happened during the Boer War when 40% of volunteers were physically unfit. However, only a small change was brought in after the Boer War with some workers being given health insurance. On the other hand, Beveridge's report put a lot of pressure on the government, which was influential in setting up the NHS. Without Beveridge's report and the efforts of Aneurin Bevan, the government may not have created the NHS.

Page 61 — The Government's Role in Healthcare

Knowledge and Understanding

1 a) The government ran a vaccination campaign from 1940 and publicised their campaign using posters, newspaper advertisements and radio broadcasts.
   b) A vaccine was introduced. They also ran a national campaign that aimed to vaccinate every person under the age of 40.
   c) The government launched the Drinkaware campaign, which included putting the Drinkaware logo on alcohol advertisements.

2   You can choose any option, so long as you explain your answer. For example:
The diphtheria campaign was the most successful. It reduced the number of cases from 60,000 in 1940 (when the campaign was launched), down to 38 in 1957. The death toll also dropped in this time, from 3,000 down to 6. While the polio campaign also reduced the number of cases, the drop wasn't as significant as the diphtheria campaign. Although the Drinkaware campaign has caused drinking to fall, it is still a lifestyle factor that leads to disease, suggesting the Drinkaware campaign hasn't been as successful as the diphtheria campaign.

Answers

3   Before the NHS, the easiest way to vaccinate children between the ages of 5-15 years old was in schools. The NHS allowed children to be vaccinated before their first birthday.

Thinking Historically

1   Jenner showed that disease could be prevented through vaccination when he introduced the smallpox vaccination. This has led to numerous other vaccinations being created, including ones for diphtheria and polio.

2 a)   • At the beginning of the 19th century the government didn't get involved in healthcare as it was run in a laissez-faire style.
- Gave Jenner funding to open a clinic so his smallpox vaccination could be given to the public.
- Introduced the Public Health Act of 1875, which improved the hygiene of streets, kept water supplies clean and ensured the maintenance of sewerage systems to prevent cholera outbreaks.
- Introduced the 1876 River Pollution Prevention Act to stop people dumping sewage in rivers. This helped to prevent diseases, such as cholera, infecting drinking water.

  b) • British and American governments encouraged businesses to mass-produce penicillin for World War II, which eventually led to its general use.
- Set up the NHS in 1948, which provided free healthcare.
- Ran publicity campaigns to encourage people to get vaccinated against diseases like diphtheria and polio.
- Passed laws to try to reduce air pollution, which causes breathing conditions like asthma and bronchitis.

  c) • Ran the Change4Life campaign which promoted daily exercise and healthy diets to combat obesity.
- Ran the Drinkaware campaign to encourage people to reduce their alcohol intake in order to decrease the cases of liver cirrhosis.

3   You can choose any option, as long as you explain your answer. For example:
The government had the biggest effect on healthcare in the 19th century. The introduction of the 1875 Public Health Act meant that sewerage systems and water supplies were properly maintained, which dramatically reduced cases of cholera. Prior to this, cholera epidemics had killed tens of thousands of people, so these measures had a huge impact on public healthcare.

4   Here are some points you may include:
- The introduction of the NHS was the most important development in British medicine during c.1900-present. The NHS provides the British public with free healthcare, making treatment accessible to even the poorest members of society. Prior to the NHS, some members of society couldn't afford to see doctors or buy medicine. The NHS has given everyone in society access to effective healthcare.
- The discovery of penicillin was the most important development in British medicine during c.1900-present. It prevented many deaths from infection during World War II, and it is used to treat a number of bacterial infections such as chest infections and skin infections. Penicillin has also paved the way for numerous other antibiotics, which can be used to treat diseases such as lung infections and meningitis.

- The discovery of viruses was the most important development in British medicine during c.1900-present. Beijerinck's work showed that viruses couldn't be treated using antibiotics in the same way that bacterial infections can be. Therefore, the discovery of viruses led to the development of antiviral drugs, which prevent a viral infection from growing.

Page 63 — Case Study: Lung Cancer

Knowledge and Understanding

1   Richard Doll and Austin Bradford Hill

2   Any three of the following:
- Chest X-rays show if there's anything on the lung that isn't usually there. This can inform doctors that they need to investigate potential signs of lung cancer.
- CT scans are used to give a more in-depth image of the lungs.
- Bronchoscopies are used to diagnose lung cancer, by putting a thin tube into the lungs to take a sample of cells.
- Modern surgery means the affected lung can be removed.
- Radiotherapy treats lung cancer by directing radiation at the lung.
- Chemotherapy uses drugs which are normally directed into the bloodstream to treat lung cancer.

3   • 1962 — Royal College of Physicians recommends a ban on tobacco advertising.
- 1965 — Cigarette adverts are banned from television.
- 1971 — Tobacco companies are forced to put health warnings on cigarette packets.
- 2007 — The government bans smoking in public places in England and Wales.
- 2015 — Parliament passes a law that requires cigarette companies to use plain packaging on cigarette boxes.

Thinking Historically

1   Similarities:
In both cases, the government responded to the discoveries by becoming more active in improving public health. After John Snow's discovery, the government introduced the 1875 Public Health Act and the 1876 River Pollution Act to reduce further outbreaks of cholera. Similarly, since Doll and Bradford Hill's discovery, the government has been active in trying to encourage a decline in smoking by introducing legislation such as banning cigarette adverts on television in 1965 and banning smoking in public places in 2007.
Differences:
Doll and Bradford Hill's discovery about the link between smoking and lung cancer was accepted when it was published in 1950. However, Snow's discovery was met with more sceptical responses because it wasn't fully proved until the Germ Theory was published in 1861.

2   You can choose either option, so long as you explain your answer. For example:
John Snow's discovery of the link between cholera and contaminated water prompted the biggest government response because it required the government to take its first big role in healthcare. Before this, the government had a laissez-faire attitude to public health so they didn't intervene in healthcare issues. However, Snow's discovery led to the government taking action and introducing the 1875 Public Health Act. This act created great change in Britain, and led to better healthcare in towns and cities.

Answers

3 Cure disease:
- Matinus Beijernick — his discovery led to the development of antiviral drugs to help cure viruses.
- Alexander Fleming — tried to find a cure to staphylococcal and discovered penicillin. This also led to the development of other antibiotics which are used to cure disease.
- Paul Ehrlich — found a cure for syphilis with the first magic bullet, Salvarsan 606.
- Gerhard Domagk — cured streptococcus with the second magic bullet, Prontosil.
- Government — through Bevan, they introduced the NHS which improved access to healthcare, allowing many people to be cured of disease.

Prevent disease:
- Government — led national vaccination campaigns to prevent diphtheria and polio.
- Government — led lifestyle campaigns such as Change4Life and Drinkaware to prevent disease.
- Government — passed a law to limit air pollution to prevent deaths from breathing conditions such as asthma and bronchitis.
- Government — banned smoking in public places, ran campaigns on helping people to give up smoking, and passed a law requiring cigarette companies to use plain boxes to prevent lung cancer.

4 You can choose either option, so long as you explain your answer. For example:
Since c.1900, there has been more emphasis on preventing disease than curing disease, especially in the second half of the 20th century. Discoveries about the cures for diseases, such as Fleming's work on penicillin and Ehrlich's work on magic bullets, came at the start of 20th century. More recently, government campaigns, such as Change4Life and Drinkaware, have focused on promoting lifestyle changes in order to prevent disease.

Pages 66-67 — Exam-Style Questions

1 This question is level marked. You should look at the level descriptions on page 85 to help you mark your answer. Here are some points your answer may include:
- In both periods, individuals put pressure on the government to improve healthcare. In 1855, John Snow published a report which established a link between cholera and contaminated water. His work was an important factor in the government creating the 1875 Public Health Act, which required councils to maintain sewerage systems to prevent further cholera outbreaks. In 1942, William Beveridge published a report which called for more government involvement in healthcare, and gained support from the public. This support put pressure on the Labour government to establish the NHS in 1948.
- In both periods, the government funded successful vaccination campaigns. In 1802, the government gave Edward Jenner £10,000 to open a clinic to vaccinate people against smallpox. The campaign was a success, and the number of cases of smallpox fell. During the 1900s, the government funded national campaigns to encourage people to get the diphtheria vaccine. By 1957, the number of diphtheria cases was just 38.

- In both periods, the government increased the accessibility of hospital care. During the 1800s, the government increased the number of hospitals, and they ensured that access to hospitals improved for both rich and poor patients. In 1948, the government formed the NHS which gave free and more accessible healthcare to everyone in Britain, including the use of hospital services.

2 This question is level marked. You should look at the level descriptions on page 85 to help you mark your answer. Here are some points your answer may include:
- New scientific discoveries led to improvements in surgery from the end of the 19th century. Landsteiner's discovery of blood groups in 1900 meant that blood transfusions became more successful. This led to fewer people dying as a result of blood loss during surgery. During World War I, doctors discovered that sodium citrate stopped blood from clotting. This improved surgery since it meant that blood could be stored outside the body so it could be available for surgeons when they needed it.
- Improved technology made surgery safer and more efficient. Robot-assisted surgery was widely used by the end of the twentieth century — it changed how surgery was performed. It allows surgeons to make smaller cuts, which leads to less scarring and a smaller risk of infection. Improvements to X-rays, which are used to examine internal disease which may require surgery, have changed in the way they're carried out. In 1904, people had to swallow or be injected with a dye so organs showed up on the X-ray, but this was no longer the case by the end of the 20th century.
- The discovery of immunosuppressants in the second half of the 20th century reduced the chance of organ rejection. This meant organ transplants could be carried out with a higher level of success.
- The work of individuals changed surgery. Christiaan Barnard performed the first successful heart transplant in 1967. This showed that it could be successfully done and furthered the research into transplants.
- The introduction of the NHS in 1948 has changed surgery. The NHS provides free healthcare, including surgical procedures. The means that surgery is now much more common and accessible for more people.

3 This question is level marked. You should look at the level descriptions on page 85 to help you mark your answer. Here are some points your answer may include:
- Fleming's discovery was the most important moment in medicine, as it showed that bacterial diseases could be treated. Pasteur and Koch had proven that bacteria caused disease towards the end of the 19th century, but no one had found a way to treat these bacteria. The discovery of penicillin confirmed that bacterial infections could be treated.
- Fleming's work led to further antibiotics being discovered. These are still used today to treat diseases such as lung infections and bacterial meningitis. These life-saving treatments might not exist without Fleming's discovery of penicillin.
- The American and British governments recognised the importance of penicillin in the 1940s. They funded the mass production of penicillin which allowed it to be used on the front lines by medics which saved the lives of countless soldiers.

Answers

- Although Fleming discovered penicillin, he wasn't able to purify it or get funding to continue his research. The work of Florey and Chain helped get penicillin to the mass market and arguably contributed more to the success of penicillin than Fleming.
- The formation of the NHS was the most important moment in medicine since c.1900. It made healthcare more accessible for ordinary people. This revolutionised the healthcare system and led to a general improvement in the public's health.
- Ivanovsky and Beijernick's discovery of viruses identified another cause of disease. This led to research into the treatment of viruses and the development of antiviral drugs.
- The discovery of DNA by Crick and Watson in 1953 showed that diseases also could be caused by genetic conditions. This has led to improved knowledge of how to diagnose and treat genetic diseases, using techniques like gene therapy.
- The discovery of magic bullets in the first half of the 20th century showed that synthetic antibodies could be used to treat disease. The development of synthetic antibodies has contributed to the growth of the pharmaceutical industry, which mass-produces medication on a large scale. This industry has made life-saving drugs cheaper and more readily available.

4 This question is level marked. You should look at the level descriptions on page 85 to help you mark your answer. Here are some points your answer may include:
- The purpose of hospitals in the 20th century was different to the purpose of hospitals in the medieval period. In the 20th century, the main purpose of hospitals was to treat disease and injury. In the medieval period, the main purpose of hospitals was to provide food, water and a warm place to stay, rather than to treat disease.
- The range of technology and treatments available to patients in 20th century hospitals was greater than those offered by hospitals in the medieval period. Hospitals in the 20th century offered advanced technology like robot-assisted surgery, and treatments like penicillin. Hospitals in the medieval period had good water and sewerage systems, but lacked the technology and treatments available to 20th century hospitals.
- Since 1948, most hospitals in Britain have been run by the National Health Service, which is supported by the government. In the medieval period, most hospitals were set up and run by the Catholic Church, which meant there was a focus on spiritual and religious healing rather than treatments based on science.

5 This question is level marked. You should look at the level descriptions on page 85 to help you mark your answer. Here are some points your answer may include:
- Ideas around the causes of disease have changed as people have developed a better understanding of disease. For example, Crick and Watson's discovery of DNA in 1953 showed that disease can also be caused by faulty genes. This led to greater understanding about genetic diseases like haemophilia. Also, the discovery of viruses in 1898 showed that diseases weren't just caused by bacteria. Beijernick found that viruses had different properties to bacteria and therefore required a different treatment. Breakthroughs such as these have helped promote the idea that causes of disease are complex, and that one theory can't explain the cause of every disease.

- People in Britain are more aware of how to change their lifestyle to improve their health. Before the 20th century, having a healthy lifestyle had been suggested as a way to prevent illness but the link between lifestyle factors and illness had never been proven. In the 20th century, scientists found that, for example, a poor diet could lead to obesity which could cause heart conditions.
- During the 20th century, it became easier to spread information, so that other scientists and the general public are more aware of the causes of disease. For example, Doll and Bradford Hill proved that smoking can cause lung cancer in 1950. Since the publication of their findings, the government has used campaigns and advertising to increase awareness about the dangers of smoking.
- Technological advancements meant that it has become easier to investigate diseases. For example, the development of CT scans in 1972 gave doctors a more detailed picture of what's going inside a patient's body. This allowed doctors and scientists to better understand the causes of disease.

6 This question is level marked. You should look at the level descriptions on page 85 to help you mark your answer. Here are some points your answer may include:
- In the 19th century, the government played an important role in improving public health. The 1875 Public Health Act was the first compulsory government intervention in public health and was effective in improving towns' water and sewerage systems. The government also supported major projects to improve public health like the Artisans' Dwelling Act.
- In the 19th and 20th centuries, the government played an important role in preventing disease. In 1802, Parliament supported Jenner's smallpox vaccine with a £10,000 grant, and in 1853 the government made the vaccination compulsory for infants. In the early 20th century, the Liberal government introduced the National Insurance Act, which gave some workers health insurance. The government also funded campaigns in the 20th century to prevent diseases caused by obesity, smoking and excessive alcohol consumption.
- In the 20th century, the government played an important role in improving public health, as it significantly improved access to medical treatment. In 1948, the government established the National Health Service, which has improved people's health by offering a range of medical services free of charge.
- Other factors were more important in improving public health before the 19th century, as the government then believed in a laissez-faire approach towards public health. This did not begin to change until the government granted funding to Jenner's smallpox vaccination clinic in the early 19th century.
- During the medieval period, the Church was more important than the government in improving people's health, as it was monasteries that ran most hospitals and tried to provide care for the poor, sick and elderly.
- In the Renaissance period, the advancement of medical knowledge played a more important role than the government. For example, Sydenham's work on the classification of diseases (e.g. showing that scarlet fever was different to measles) helped doctors to diagnose diseases more easily.

Answers

- The development of technology like the printing press in the 1470s was also significant, as it allowed new medical ideas to be spread more easily. This helped to disprove old ideas about medicine. For example, the printing press allowed many people to read Vesalius' ideas about dissection and anatomy, which questioned Galen and encouraged others to challenge his ideas.
- In many cases, government action to improve people's health only came about because of advances in science and technology. For example, after Pasteur's Germ Theory was published in 1861, the link between poor living conditions and poor health became more widely accepted. The Germ Theory provided the scientific proof required to persuade the government to pass the 1875 Public Health Act.

The British Sector of the Western Front, 1914-1918

Page 69 — Trench Warfare on the Western Front

Source Analysis

1 a) The content of Source A is useful because it suggests that hospitals struggled to cope with the number of injured soldiers during the Battle of the Somme. Tens of thousands of soldiers were injured in the first week of the battle, and the author of the source reveals that her hospital didn't have enough space to treat everyone who was brought to it.

b) Source A is useful because it was written by a nurse who cared for injured soldiers during the Battle of the Somme. This means that she would have had a good idea about how well equipped the medical staff were to treat injured soldiers, so the information she provides is likely to be reliable. However, the usefulness of the source is limited because the author can only tell us about the provision of medical care when the soldiers had reached hospital — it doesn't tell us how well prepared the British Army was for treating soldiers closer to the front line.

c) Source A is useful because it was written during the Battle of the Somme, so it is likely to be an accurate record of the author's experience of the shortage of beds in the hospital. However, the usefulness of the source is limited because the diary entry was written just a few days after the beginning of the battle. This means that it doesn't show whether medical provision improved as the fighting continued or whether the shortage of beds continued to be a problem.

2 a) Source B shows a large number of wounded men waiting on stretchers to be taken to hospital. During the Battle of the Somme, an enormous number of men were wounded — there were almost 60,000 British casualties in the first week of the battle alone. The source is useful because it indicates that these high casualty numbers had an impact on the provision of medical care, forcing many men to wait in the open air rather than being immediately taken to hospital and treated.

b) Source B is a photograph. This makes it useful, because it should be an accurate representation of the scene — with so many men involved, it is unlikely to have been staged. However, Source B's usefulness is limited because, as a photograph, it only provides information about one specific place and time. It can't give us any information about how long the wounded men had to wait before and after the picture was taken, or about the sort of medical care that was available once they were transferred to hospital.

Knowledge and Understanding

1
- The British Army used mines to break through the enemy lines at Arras and Ypres in 1917. This was intended to weaken the defences of enemy trenches and reduce casualties among infantry.
- The British Army set up more medical posts before major offensives to make sure the injured could be treated more quickly. For example, there were 379 Medical Officers at the Third Battle of Ypres in late 1917, compared to 174 during the first week of the Battle of the Somme.
- The British Army set up a blood bank at the Battle of Cambrai. This made it easier to save lives during the battle because there was a supply of blood available.

2
- Entrenching — Lots of soldiers in a line would dig straight into the ground.
- Sapping — One soldier would dig outwards from the end of a trench.
- Tunnelling — One soldier would dig outwards from the end of a trench, but leave a layer of earth on top of the trench until it was finished.

3
- Parados — A mound of earth or sandbags that raised the height of the back of the trench to protect soldiers from shell explosions behind the trench.
- Duckboards — Wooden boards used to line the floors of trenches in wet areas.
- Parapet — A mound of earth on the front side of the trench lined with wooden planks, netting or sandbags. It was designed to be bulletproof to protect soldiers.
- Firing step — A step in fire trenches where soldiers would stand to fire their rifles over the parapet and into no man's land.
- Barbed wire — Set in front of the trench to make it harder for the enemy to attack.
- No man's land — The ground between the front line trenches of each side.

Page 71 — Trench Warfare on the Western Front

Knowledge and Understanding

1
- Saps — Small trenches that pushed out of the front line into no man's land.
- The fire trench — A trench on the front line that faced the enemy directly, so that soldiers could fire at them. The fire trench had zig-zags or step-shaped sections separated by traverses to contain explosions and to stop enemy infantry from firing along the trench.
- The supervision trench — Another trench on the front line, immediately behind the fire trench. It had a similar shape to the fire trench, and was used to move along the front line.

Answers

- The support trench — The support trench reinforced the front line and soldiers could retreat to it. It was protected from shell bombardment aimed at the front line, but was connected to the front line by communication trenches.
- Communication trenches — Used to connect different trench lines to each other, as well as to roads and army depots behind the lines.
- The reserve trench — Situated about 350-550 metres behind the front line. It was made up of dugouts or lines of trenches. Reinforcements would wait here.

2
- At Arras, the Allies built a tunnel network by extending existing caves, quarries and mines. Before the Battle of Arras, the tunnel network was used to hide 24,000 men. Tunnellers dug up to the German line, then used mines to blow open the entrances. This allowed the Allies to reach the German trenches in safety.
- At the Battle of Messines, 19 mines were blown up under the German line. They killed around 10,000 German soldiers and destroyed German defences on Hill 60 and the Caterpillar, making the German position easier to attack.

3   It was difficult to evacuate wounded men from the front lines quickly because trench warfare damaged roads and terrain, making it hard for motor and horse-drawn vehicles to move around. Instead, stretcher bearers had to evacuate men on foot along communication trenches or through relay posts.

4   It became easier for the British Army to evacuate wounded men by 1917 because a railway network was built behind the lines, which could move men more quickly across the muddy, damaged terrain.

Source Analysis

1 a) • Why did injured soldiers have to wait for transport?
- An official military record of the number of motor and horse-drawn vehicles made available by the British Army at the Battle of Arras.
- This would show whether a lack of vehicles was a factor in why there was limited transport to and from the front line.

b) • How badly did the Battle of Arras affect the local transport infrastructure?
- Some aerial photographs of the battlefield and the surrounding area taken before and after the battle.
- This would show the extent to which the roads in the local area were damaged by the fighting.

c) • How far did stretcher bearers have to walk to reach transport?
- The diaries of men who worked as stretcher bearers at the Battle of Arras.
- This would show the distance that stretcher bearers had to travel to reach transport, showing how difficult it was to evacuate wounded men from the front quickly.

Page 73 — The RAMC and the FANY

Source Analysis

1 b) How easy was it for injured soldiers to find dressing stations?
c) Was it common for dressing stations to be in such a poor condition?
d) How well staffed were dressing stations?

2 a) An official record of the number of stretcher bearers at the Third Battle of Ypres would show whether a lack of stretcher bearers stopped injured soldiers from being moved away from the front line in an efficient way.

b) A map of the Third Battle of Ypres showing the location of the dressing stations in the area would show how far from the front line injured soldiers had to travel to get to the nearest one.

c) Some photographs of other British dressing stations from around that time would help to establish whether the one Sherriff visited was typical, or whether other dressing stations were in better condition.

d) An RAMC record of the number of medical staff in different Field Ambulance units, their qualifications, and where they were posted would show how well staffed each dressing station was. It would also show whether the staff at dressing stations always included highly-trained professionals such as doctors and nurses.

Knowledge and Understanding

1 a) Regimental Aid Posts — These gave first aid to soldiers a few metres behind the front line.
b) Dressing Stations — These collected injured men from the Regimental Aid Posts using horse-drawn ambulances and stretcher bearers, and gave them basic medical treatment.
c) Casualty Clearing Stations — These collected seriously injured men from the Dressing Stations using convoys of motor ambulances. They had medical staff (including nurses) who treated men for up to four weeks before sending them back to the Front or to a Base Hospital.
d) Base Hospitals — These treated common injuries and ailments, such as the effects of gas. They treated men until they could be sent back to the Front or sent home to Britain.

2 a) The RAMC were responsible for setting up medical stations and moving casualties between them. Their Field Ambulance units used stretcher bearers, horse-drawn ambulances and motor ambulances to move casualties between medical stations, or to take them somewhere they could be moved more quickly and easily (e.g. by road, rail or river).

b) The FANY mostly worked as a field ambulance, moving casualties between hospitals, medical stations or even coastal ports where they could be taken back to Britain. The FANY also staffed hospitals, as well as providing other services for the troops including a canteen, soup kitchen and bathing vehicle.

Page 75 — Conditions in the Trenches

Knowledge and Understanding

1 a) Frostbite was caused by exposure to the cold.
b) Soldiers got trench foot by standing in flooded trenches for too long.
c) Dysentery was the main cause of diarrhoea and dehydration, and the disease spread quickly in the trenches due to dirty water and unhygienic latrines.
d) The trenches were full of disease-spreading body lice which carried trench fever and typhus.
e) Shell shock was either a physical injury caused by damage to the central nervous system as a result of an explosion, or a psychological illness caused by the emotional trauma of living in the trenches.

2
- Lachrimatory Gas (1914) — Also known as tear gas. It caused inflammation of the nose, throat and lungs, as well as blindness. This disabled soldiers and forced them to retreat, but didn't kill them.
- Chlorine Gas (April 1915) — The first deadly gas to be used on the Western Front. It killed soldiers by slowly suffocating them.

Answers

Answers

- Phosgene (December 1915) — This gas also suffocated soldiers, but it was odourless and colourless to make it harder to detect. The symptoms could take more than 24 hours to set in.
- Mustard Gas (July 2017) — A 'blistering agent', which caused blisters, burns and breathing difficulties. It ate away at the body from the inside, meaning that it could take someone up to five weeks to die from mustard gas exposure. It also clung to the soldiers' clothes, putting medical staff at risk too.

Source Analysis

1   Investigation c) — The source is a medical case record, so it gives a clear, factual account of the patient's symptoms. For example, it describes how the patient suffered from memory loss, shakiness and headaches. This makes it very useful for an investigation into the symptoms of shell shock.

2   • The source would be less useful for Investigation a) because it describes the patient's symptoms, but doesn't go into any detail about the treatment that he received or how effective it was.
   • The source would be less useful for Investigation b) because people's understanding of shell shock changed throughout the war, and the source was written in 1915. It therefore can't provide information about the situation at the end of the war in 1918.

Page 77 — Wounds and Injuries

Knowledge and Understanding

1 a) • Trenches protected the body, but left soldiers' heads and faces exposed.
   • Soldiers received head and facial injuries as a result of enemy gunfire (e.g. machine guns and rifles).
   • Many head and facial injuries were caused by shell explosions, as well as the flying shrapnel and debris that they produced.
 b) • Cuts and bruises
   • Fractures
   • Gunshot wounds
   • Shrapnel wounds
   • Concussion
   • Brain damage
 c) • In 1915, soldiers were issued with metal 'Brodie' helmets, giving them a better chance of surviving head and facial injuries.
   • Dr Harvey Cushing developed the technique of using X-rays to locate shrapnel in the brain, before taking it out using magnets. This halved the number of deaths caused by brain surgery during the war.
   • Dr Harold Gillies developed a plastic surgery technique known as the tube pedicle, making the treatment of serious facial injuries more effective.

2   • Many trenches were dug in farmland, which was covered in bacteria from fertilisers. The fact that the trenches were often waterlogged allowed these bacteria to thrive.
   • The ground was infected by unhygienic latrines, as well as dead bodies that were left to decompose or buried in shallow graves.
   • Many wounded soldiers had to lie in contaminated mud for hours or days before stretcher bearers were able to take them away, leaving them vulnerable to infections.

3 a) Given to soldiers on the front line to prevent tetanus.
 b) Used to wash soldiers' wounds before they were bandaged.
 c) Used on open wounds to cover them up and protect them from infection.
 d) Used to prevent the spread of life-threatening infections from the arms, legs, hands or feet to the rest of the body.

Source Analysis

1 a) The source is useful because it was written by a member of medical staff at a hospital in Newcastle, where injured soldiers were treated after returning to England. Therefore, the author would have had a good understanding of the treatment of head injuries, so the information the source contains is likely to be reliable. However, the usefulness of the source is limited because the author wasn't directly involved in treating the soldier on the Western Front. This means that the information the author provides is based on the patient's account of the treatment they received — the patient's memory of their treatment might not be completely accurate because of the serious head injury they had suffered.
 b) The source is useful because it was written on 26 July 1915, not long after the patient suffered a gunshot wound to the head (9 July 1915). It is therefore likely to be an accurate record of the main events in the patient's treatment. However, the two-week gap between the injury and the writing of the source means that it may not contain the same level of detail as a source written immediately after the events described.
 c) The purpose of the source is to record the medical treatment received by the patient. This makes it useful because it would have been important for the information in the medical case records to be accurate. However, the source is only meant to record the treatment of a single patient, so other medical case records would need to be studied to build up an overall impression of the treatment of head injuries on the Western Front.
 d) The content of the source is useful because it shows that the medical staff at Casualty Clearing Stations were able to perform surgery on patients who had suffered serious head injuries before sending them to hospital. It also suggests that the medical staff who performed surgery were concerned about the risk of infection and sepsis and took measures to avoid them. However, it doesn't provide many specific details about how the operation was carried out, or how the patient was treated afterwards.

Page 79 — Developments in Surgery and Medicine

Knowledge and Understanding

1 a) • Delayed primary closure
   • To prevent and treat wound infection
   • The wound was explored thoroughly to remove any shrapnel, clothing or damaged tissue. It was washed with antiseptic, before being left open to the air for 24 to 48 hours. The wound was then checked for bacteria by looking at a swab under a microscope. It was only closed up at this stage if it wasn't infected.
 b) • Irrigation
   • To prevent and treat wound infection
   • The wound was flushed out with an antiseptic solution using rubber tubes before closure.

Answers

c) • Thomas splint
   • To treat a fractured femur.
   • The splint was strapped around the broken leg to stop it from moving. This protected the leg from more damage.

2   X-ray machines meant that surgeons didn't have to look for shrapnel and bone fragments by hand. This reduced the chance of wounds becoming infected. The development of mobile X-ray units meant that soldiers could be treated closer to the front line.

3 a) The syringe-cannula technique was developed. Doctors took blood from a donor using a needle and syringe, which allowed the blood to be transfused more quickly.

b) In 1914, sodium citrate started to be added to blood so that it could be stored without clotting. In 1916, blood started to be added to a citrate glucose solution, allowing it to be stored on ice for 10 to 14 days.

c) At the Battle of Cambrai in 1917, a blood bank was set up to collect blood before it was needed.

Source Analysis

1   The source is useful because it was published towards the end of the war in June 1918, by which point a lot of progress had already been made in solving the problem of blood loss on the Western Front. Developments such as using sodium citrate to stop blood from clotting meant that blood could be stored, and the source shows that by 1918 medical experts were confident that stored blood was just as effective as fresh blood. However, the source doesn't tell us how the problem of blood loss was tackled before blood could be stored.

2   The source was written by Captain Oswald Robertson, who was a surgeon in the US Army. In 1917, he set up the first blood bank in preparation for the Battle of Cambrai. He is therefore an expert witness on the problem of blood loss on the Western Front. This gives authority to the information that Robertson provides about the effectiveness of using stored blood.

Page 81 — Types of Sources
Knowledge and Understanding

1 a) • Medical records, official reports by the Royal Army Medical Corps and army officers, hospital admission records, government reports.
   • Documents can be useful if you're looking for factual information about a historical site or the people who used it. There's often a date attached, which is useful if you're looking for evidence from a specific point in a site's history. Some documents (e.g. official records) also help to spot patterns or to understand how typical a piece of evidence is.
   • It's sometimes hard to judge how reliable the facts in documents are. This is because they're usually quite one-sided and it's not always clear who wrote them.

b) • Diaries, memoirs, first-hand reports, autobiographies, oral accounts.
   • First-hand accounts are useful for finding out what it was like to live and work at a particular site because they provide details that less personal sources (e.g. documents) don't mention.
   • First-hand accounts are so personal that they're only useful as evidence for the experiences of the people who wrote them. First-hand accounts that were written a long time after the events they describe might contain inaccuracies because the author may have forgotten details or focused on some details more than others.

c) • Photographs, maps, plans, diagrams, artwork.
   • Photographs show what a historical site looked like at a particular time, while maps, plans and diagrams help to work out how the site was laid out and organised. They can cover large areas to put a site into its wider context or focus on a specific feature of a site to give a detailed picture of how it looked and worked.
   • Images don't always provide a full picture. For example, the photographer can choose what to focus on and what to leave out of a photograph. They could even stage a photograph in order to show an idealised version of a historical site and the people who used it.

Source Analysis

1 a) Were Field Ambulance units affected by gas attacks?
  b) Did all Field Ambulance units use the same evacuation procedure?
  c) Were head injuries common among members of Field Ambulance units?
  d) How quickly were new techniques such as the Thomas splint adopted by Field Ambulance units?

2 a) An official photo of another Field Ambulance unit from a different part of the Western Front. If there were gas masks in the photo, it would indicate that other units were also at risk of experiencing gas attacks.
  b) The training schedules of other Field Ambulance units would allow us to see whether all units received the same training, or whether there were any major differences. This would give us a good impression of whether or not all Field Ambulance units would have followed the same evacuation procedure.
  c) A set of hospital admission records for a base hospital near to where the 44th Field Ambulance operated would reveal whether any of the patients were members of the 44th Field Ambulance, and what their injuries were. This would help to establish whether or not head injuries were common in the 44th Field Ambulance.
  d) The medical case records for injured soldiers returning to England would provide information about how they were treated on the Western Front. This would give us an impression of when Field Ambulance units started to use new techniques such as the Thomas splint to treat injured soldiers.

Page 84 — Exam-Style Questions

1   Each feature is marked separately and you can have a maximum of two marks per feature. How to grade your answer:
   • 1 mark for describing one credible feature of Base Hospitals on the Western Front.
   • 2 marks for describing one feature and for giving some supporting information that provides more detail.
   Here are some points your answer may include:
   • Base Hospitals were the last location in the Chain of Evacuation, furthest away from the front line. They treated patients until they could be sent back to the Front or sent home to Britain.
   • Base Hospitals were established in large buildings. They could take up to 400 patients.
   • Base Hospitals were often turned into specialist hospitals. They might specialise in common injuries and health problems, such as the effects of gas attacks.
   • Base Hospitals were often set up near transport networks. This made it easier for medical units to move injured soldiers to and from hospital.

Answers

- Base Hospitals had X-ray machines. These were used to detect broken bones and shrapnel.

2   This question is level marked. You should look at the level descriptions below to help you mark your answer.

8-mark questions:

Level 1 1-2 marks	The answer gives a simple analysis of the sources to come to a basic judgement about their usefulness for the investigation. It shows a basic understanding of the sources' content and/or provenance, as well as displaying some relevant knowledge of the topic.
Level 2 3-5 marks	The answer analyses the sources in more detail to make judgements about their usefulness for the investigation. It shows a good understanding of the sources' content and/or provenance and uses relevant knowledge to support its judgements.
Level 3 6-8 marks	The answer evaluates the sources to make judgements about their usefulness for the investigation. It shows a detailed understanding of the sources and uses relevant knowledge to analyse their content and provenance, and to support its judgements.

Here are some points your answer may include:
- Source A is useful because it describes several different symptoms of shell shock, such as sleeplessness and depression. We know that the impact of trench warfare on soldiers could be severe. This is supported by the details given in the source.
- Source A is useful because Rivers was a psychiatrist who had experience working with shell-shocked soldiers from the Western Front. He can therefore be regarded an expert witness, which gives credibility to the medical detail the source contains about the impact of trench warfare on soldiers' mental health.
- Source A's usefulness is limited because, as a psychiatrist, Rivers focuses solely on the impact of trench warfare on soldiers' mental health. The source doesn't provide any information about the physical health problems caused by trench warfare.
- Source A's usefulness is limited by the fact that it only describes how trench warfare affected one soldier. It would be necessary to study the experiences of many different soldiers to develop a more general picture of the impact of trench warfare on soldiers on the Western Front.
- Source B is useful because it reveals the impact of gas attacks by showing many soldiers with bandages over their eyes. Gas attacks could lead to severe health problems such as blindness, and this is supported by the source.
- Source B is useful because it suggests that gas attacks were a part of trench warfare that could hurt many soldiers. In the image, a large group of men have been injured by a gas attack, which shows that gas attacks could have a devastating impact on lots of soldiers at once.

- The usefulness of Source B is limited because it is a painting. Although we know that the artist experienced life on the battlefield, we can't be sure that the event portrayed in the picture actually took place. Sargent might also have been selective about what details to include or leave out. For example, in the painting the ground is in good condition and there isn't much mud, but we know that damaged, muddy terrain was a very common problem on the Western Front.
- Source B's usefulness is limited because the artist was sponsored by the British government. It is likely that the government influenced the content of Sargent's painting so that it would convey a particular message to the public. This means that we cannot be sure that the painting accurately shows the impact of trench warfare.

3   How to grade your answer:
   a) 1 mark for giving a detail from Source A that you could investigate.
   b) 1 mark for giving a question you would ask to further investigate the detail from Source A.
   c) 1 mark for suggesting an appropriate source to use.
   d) 1 mark for explaining how the source would help to answer your follow-up question.

For example:
   a) 'the most terrible depression'
   b) Was depression a common symptom among soldiers suffering from shell shock?
   c) A set of medical case records from a hospital specialising in the treatment of shell shock.
   d) The medical case records would help me to find out how common depression was among sufferers of shell shock, and whether it was more or less common than the other symptoms.

Index